Clinics in Developmental Medicine No. 148
THE NEUROLOGICAL ASSESSMENT
OF THE PRETERM AND FULL-TERM
NEWBORN INFANT

Senior Editor: Martin C.O. Bax
Editor: Hilary M. Hart
Managing Editor: Michael Pountney
Sub Editor: Suzanne Miller

Set in Times and Avant Garde on QuarkXPress

First edition 1981
Second edition 1999

British Library Cataloguing-in-Publication data:
A catalogue record for this book is available from the British Library

ISSN: 0069 4835
ISBN: 1 898683 15 8

Originally printed by The Lavenham Press Ltd, Water Street, Lavenham, Suffolk

Clinics in Developmental Medicine No. 148

The Neurological Assessment of the Preterm & Full-term Newborn Infant

2nd Edition

LILLY MS DUBOWITZ
VICTOR DUBOWITZ
EUGENIO MERCURI

Department of Paediatrics and Neonatal Medicine
Hammersmith Hospital
Postgraduate Medical School
London

1999
Mac Keith Press

AUTHORS' APPOINTMENTS

Lilly M S Dubowitz MD, FRCP, FRCPH — Honorary Senior Lecturer in Paediatrics, Imperial College School of Medicine, London, UK

Victor Dubowitz, MD, PhD, FRCP, FRCPH — Emeritus Professor of Paediatrics, Imperial College School of Medicine, London, UK

Eugenio Mercuri, MD, PhD — Lecturer in Paediatric Neurology, Imperial College School of Medicine, London, UK

The newborn infant may be described as a tonic animal with oropharyngeal and other automatisms and neuro-vegetative mechanisms.

POLANI AND MAC KEITH 1960

We have to assume that a consciousness similar to our own and therefore understandable to us does not exist in the child before the end of the first year of life.

PEIPER 1963

A thorough knowledge and understanding of the normal development of the infant and young child is just as fundamental to anyone concerned with the care of children, especially paediatricians, as is anatomy to the surgeon.

ILLINGWORTH 1960

One single examination of the newborn infant is not sufficient.

SAINT-ANNE DARGASSIES 1962

It is not difficult to compose long lists of reflexes which may be elicited from infants, or devise detailed schemata of examinations by scratching, thumping, spinning, or otherwise invading their privacy. It is a good deal harder to find signs which reliably predict lasting CNS damage.

CLARK 1964

Many experienced neurologists and investigators feel that there may never be a satisfactory neurological examination for the newborn.

PARMELEE AND MICHAELIS 1971

Paediatric neurologists are strange people. The trouble is they're not really interested in neurology, they're only interested in children.

ONE-TIME PRESIDENT OF ASSOCIATION OF BRITISH NEUROLOGISTS

It is in practice impossible to examine all newborn infants, although this might be an ideal condition, and therefore great care has been taken in identifying those infants at risk of neurological problems.

PRECHTL 1977

A difficult labour is not evidence of injury to the baby's brain, nor is a normal labour proof that the brain in unharmed.

MAC KEITH 1977

In many ways, there are greater differences between the brain of a 28 week infant and that of a 36 week infant than there are between the brain of the three-month old baby and an adult.

PAPE AND WIGGLESWORTH 1979

I am becoming more and more convinced of the importance of distinguishing that which is interesting from that which is important, and of focussing down onto tests which are relevant for assessment, while excluding those which merely take time and provide no useful information.

ILLINGWORTH 1980

Ideally, a meaningful neurological assessment should form part of the routine clinical examination of every newborn infant.

DUBOWITZ AND DUBOWITZ 1981

Handicap results from the complex interaction of many elements which affect the way in which the child comes to terms with his world.

MITCHELL 1981

CONTENTS

PREFACE TO THE SECOND EDITION

When we wrote the first edition of this book in the late 1970s, the neurological assessment of the newborn infant was, at best, still rudimentary in most neonatal units, and the non-invasive imaging techniques of the brain, initially with computer tomography and subsequently the more practical ultrasound imaging, were still in their infancy. We expressed the hope that "ideally, a meaningful neurological assessment should form part of the routine clinical examination of every newborn infant."

We have come a long way since then, and the intervening 20 years have witnessed the tremendous impact of magnetic resonance imaging of the brain, which has provided remarkable insight into the occurrence of haemorrhagic and ischaemic lesions of the newborn brain and their evolution and resolution. This has provided the opportunity of further extending the correlation of clinical signs with the site of brain lesions, as had already become possible with the advent of routine ultrasound imaging on the neonatal unit.

The neurological protocol we introduced has also found wide application, and we have tested it in many different environments, from the highly sophisticated, technology-driven, tertiary referral unit, such as our own at the Hammersmith Hospital, to several centres in the developing world. Various details have been amended and updated in the light of our experience. We have adapted the system for use in special circumstances. We have produced one simplified version for use as a practical screening tool for the routine examination of term newborn infants on the maternity unit. We have also developed a shortened and more practical version for use by local medical and paramedical staff in the rural conditions in developing countries, and this has already been extensively tested in the Karen refugee camps in northern Thailand, and in other comparable communities in central Africa. A separate chapter has been devoted to this work.

In response to many suggestions to try to quantify the system, we have developed an optimality score for each item in the assessment protocol and produced a cumulative score. This can be repeated sequentially in following the progress of an individual infant. The optimality score is intended mainly as a research tool.

We have recently also developed a comparable neurological protocol suitable for assessing infants between 2 and 24 months of age.

Hopefully, in the years to come we may still achieve our original goal of a meaningful neurological assessment as part of the routine examination of every newborn infant.

Acknowledgements
We are grateful to a number of research fellows and colleagues who have been actively involved with the development and appraisal of our updated assessment protocol over the past 18 years since the publication of the first edition. We would particularly like to thank Linda de Vries, Frances Cowan, Mary Rutherford, Deborah Murdoch-Eaton, Helen Bouza,

ix

and Juan Carlos Faundez, as well as Rivka Regev and Leena Haataja, who were involved in the development of the infant scoring system.

Thanks also to Sylvia Watson and Anne Maloy and their nursing staff on the neonatal units at Hammersmith and Queen Charlotte's hospitals for all their help and support.

We are very grateful to a number of colleagues in various malaria units abroad who helped with the evaluation and adaptation of the method to conditions in the developing world, in particular François Nosten, Director of the Shoklo Malaria Research Unit in Maesot, Thailand, and Rose McGrady and their staff; also Tharatip Kolatat and Sopapan Panavudhikrai at the Sirriraj Maternity Hospital and Julie Simpson from the Wellcome Unit at Mahidol University in Bangkok; Francine Verhoeff in Malawi; and Caroline Schulman in Kenya

We are also grateful to the Wellcome Trust for their financial support of these visits, which enabled us to develop the method for developing countries.

We would like to thank all the mothers who so readily agreed that their infants should participate in these studies.

We also wish to record our appreciation to Tom Vamos for his expertise and help with the computerization of the proformas and to Michael Dubowitz for his patience and forbearance with all the out-of-hours computer crises.

We are grateful to Michael Pountney and Suzanne Miller at MacKeith Press for their patience and forbearance with our obsession and persistence in the final layout of the manual.

LILLY DUBOWITZ, MD, FRCP, FRCPH
VICTOR DUBOWITZ, MD, PhD, FRCP, FRCPH
EUGENIO MERCURI, MD, PhD

London, October 1999

INTRODUCTION TO THE FIRST EDITION

Advances in neonatal intensive care over the past decade have revolutionized the management of severe respiratory problems in the very-low-birthweight premature infant and have considerably improved the changes of survival. Advances in management of the neurological problems of the newborn have not kept pace and intraventricular haemorrhage (IVH) is now one of the major causes of death in these premature infants. There is as yet no readily available biochemical or other window on the functional state of the nervous system comparable to that of the respiratory system. Thus it is not surprising that neonatal residents, in their zeal to maintain the homeostasis of blood gases and electrolytes, commonly lost sight of the fact that one of the main reasons for achieving optimal respiratory function is to ensure the integrity of the nervous system. Documentation of the state of the nervous sytem is usually sparse and often it may be difficult even to find information on whether the infant is alert and responsive, or comatose.

The advent of CT scanning made it possible for the first time to accurately diagnose subependymal and intraventricular haemorrhage in the premature newborn infant during life, and showed that IVH may occur in many low-birthweight infants who have no apparent clinical abnormality (Papile et al. 1978). However, CT scanning is an invasive technique, with a high ration dose for the small neonate, and is impractical and potentially hazardous for the high-risk infant who has to be moved from his intensive care environmnent to a radiology unit. Sequential ultrasound examination has now made it possible to visualize the acutal development, progression, and re solution of the germinal layer and intraventricular haemorrhage and ventricular dilatation in a newborn infant on the neonatal unit, without any disturbance ot the infant (Pape et al. 1979, Levene et al. 1981). We have to remember, however, that any imaging technique, be it CT scanning or ultrasound, at best can only reflect structural or anatomical change and cannot advise us on the functional state of the nervous system: therefore we need a clinical tool which can correlate function with these structural changes. Rational clinical management has to be based on the clinical status of the patient and not purely on aberrations revealed by technology, otherwise the treatment may prove more harmful than the disease.

The nervous system of the neonate is in a dynamic state of rapid development and any assessment of the infant has to allow not only for the possible pathological deviations but also for the state of maturity of the nervous sytem. In addition, any attempt at prognostication has to take account of the tremendous potential for resolution and compensation of the developing nervous sytem, which is probably more marked the more immature it is. It would also seem naive to assume, as has so often been done in the past, that the development of the nervous system of the infant born prematurely proceeds in the same way outside the uterus as it would have done *in utero,* as if the environment has no impact on it at all.

Ideally, a meaningful neurological assessment should form part of the routine clinical examination of every newborn infant. It should have diagnostic relevance to the detection of abnormality at the time of its occurrence in the newborn period, in the hope of identifying the causes and influencing the course and outcome of the pathological processes by timely intervention, and of preventing them in the future.

Acknowledgements

The development and standardization of this neurological scheme would not have been possible without the considerable help we have had over the years from a succession of research associates. We would particularly like to record our gratitude to the following:

Dr Adadot Hayes
Dr Rosamond Jones
Dr Marc Verghote
Dr Malcolm Levene
Dr Ana Morante
Dr Penelope Palmer
Dr Clair-Lise Fawer

1
HISTORICAL REVIEW

When we wrote the first edition of this manual in the late 1970s, we were conscious of the need for a practical scheme for the day-to-day clinical examination of the nervous system in the preterm and term newborn infant, in order to document deviant clinical signs and their evolution or resolution. That edition was not only practical, but timely, with the recent advent of new imaging techniques such as computed tomography and then ultrasound scanning and magnetic resonance imaging. The use of ultrasound imaging, in particular, for routine screening in the neonatal unit enabled us to identify haemorrhagic or ischaemic lesions in the brains of newborn infants and to correlate the clinical signs with pathological and imaging changes.

In that first edition, we acknowledged the important contribution of a number of pioneers in the previous decades, which had paved the way for the development of a neurological examination of the newborn infant. In the first part of the 20th century, Albrecht Peiper in Leipzig developed a great interest in the behaviour of the newborn infant (Peiper 1928, 1963), particularly neonatal reflexes. However, because of the similarity of some of these reflexes to those observed in pathological states in adults, or after experimental brain lesions in animals, the mistaken belief developed that the state of the young infant was similar to these pathological states. The young infant was thought to lack the functional capacity of the cortex and the cerebellum and was looked upon as a brainstem preparation, and its neural function as a bundle of reflexes. Although Peiper never developed a systematic examination for the newborn infant, he paved the way for the work of André-Thomas in Paris.

André-Thomas, who was much more interested in various aspects of muscle tone, evolved a detailed concept of different kinds of tone: *active tone,* associated with voluntary or spontaneous movements of the infant; and *passive tone,* associated with the capacity of muscles to be lengthened when joints are moved passively (extensibility) or with the resistance of muscles when distal parts of the limb are freely swung or flapped (passivity) (André-Thomas and de Ajuriaguerra 1949, André-Thomas and Saint-Anne Dargassies 1952). Saint-Anne Dargassies (1955) later developed a systematic examination of the newborn infant along these lines, and the very first volume in this series of Clinics in Developmental Medicine was devoted to a translation from the French of the neurological examination evolved by these two workers and a colleague (André-Thomas et al. 1960). In addition to the many neurological items associated with muscle tone, they also defined in detail various primitive reflexes. Mapping out the progressive maturation of these neurological features as the preterm infant develops, Saint-Anne Dargassies (1966, 1972, 1977) showed that the developmental characteristics were related to the infant's maturity (postmenstrual age), not to size. In her meticulous clinical observations, that author tried to define the gestational age at which various reflexes and responses first become apparent, and her data suggested

1

that various developmental events occur at a fixed time, with very little biological variability. She also showed that the trend in development of the infant born before term was similar outside the uterus to what normally occurs in utero. Amiel-Tison and her colleagues further developed this method of assessment by making the descriptions more objective and quantitative (Amiel-Tison 1979, Amiel-Tison and Grenier 1980). They later also included an assessment of vision and hearing (Amiel-Tison et al. 1982).

In the 1960s, Prechtl and his associates in Groningen stimulated much interest in the neurological examination of the newborn infant and considerably influenced its development (Prechtl and Dijkstra 1960, Prechtl and Beintema 1964, Beintema 1968, Prechtl 1977). They concentrated particularly on apparently normal, term infants, systematically studied the various neurological responses in the neonatal period, and tried to document objectively any deviations in these responses. They drew attention to the importance of the "state" of the infant, i.e. the degree of wakefulness or arousal, and showed the striking way in which various responses could change in relation to different states. They developed a 5-point scale for the infant's state and defined the optimal state in which to elicit various responses. Using computer analysis of deviations in individual neurological signs, they were able to recognize clustering of groups of responses and to define a number of "syndromes" on this basis. These included the "hyperexcitable" syndrome, with increased responsiveness to various stimuli; the "apathetic" syndrome, with decreased responsiveness; and the "hemisyndrome", with asymmetry of response.

Prechtl aimed to design an examination "to obtain maximum amount of information about the complex neural functions in minimum time and with no risk to the patient" (Prechtl and Beintema 1964). In the second edition of his manual (1977), Prechtl outlined the sequence of decisions necessary to design such an examination. He showed that it was necessary to standardize rigorously not only the method of eliciting the various responses but also the infant's optimal behavioural state for each component of the examination.

Prechtl's examination, which took about 30 minutes, consisted of observed and elicited items. Whenever possible, the responses were also described quantitatively or scored semi-quantitatively (by + or –). The examination was summarized under the headings posture, motility, pathological movements, motor system (abnormal tone), responses (intensity), threshold of responses, tendon reflexes, Moro response, state, cry, hemisyndrome, and syndrome of abnormal reactivity. Prechtl also devised a shorter examination suitable for screening (Prechtl 1977), consisting of a limited number of items thought to give the highest chance of differentiating between normal and suspect term infants. The items included the assessment of posture and motility in the supine position, resistance to passive movement, the traction test, sucking, the Moro response, and the position and movement of the eyes. The screening examination was found to give many more false-positive results than the full form (Touwen et al. 1977).

Prechtl's examination gave reliable information about the infant's neurological status and, when performed by experienced examiners, made it possible to differentiate between central and peripheral involvement. However, it presented various difficulties when ill infants in the neonatal unit were examined, because the findings were reliable only if the examination was performed in full, under standard conditions – both of which requirements could pose difficulties in ill infants. The examiner had to have considerable experience to be able to grade the strengths of some of the responses. All examination items chosen as most appropriate for term infants were assumed to be equally suitable for premature infants once they had reached 40 weeks postmenstrual age. There is evidence, however, that not all aspects of neuronal maturation proceed in the same way inside and outside the uterus. Thus, infants reaching 40 weeks postmenstrual age might differ from each other in accordance with their postnatal age and exposure to the extrauterine environment (Howard et al. 1976, Casaer et al. 1982, Palmer et al. 1982, Lacey et al. 1985, Piper et al. 1985).

Parmelee and Michaelis (1971) tried to devise an examination based on the Prechtl approach. They gave more explicit instructions on grading the various responses and aimed at a total score. The main shortcoming of this approach is that because some of the responses in the abnormal infant may be weaker while others are exaggerated, many abnormal infants may end up with a normal total score. It is thus not surprising that the predictive power of this examination turned out to be poor.

With the possible exception of Prechtl's evaluation of the "state" of the infant, most of the criteria in these schemes were based on tone and primitive reflexes and might thus be expected to reflect "lower" rather than "higher" neurological function. An attempt to assess higher neurological function was made by the neurobehavioural approach to the newborn infant. In the mid 1950s, Graham, a psychologist who was particularly interested in the effects of perinatal trauma and hypoxia on the newborn infant, developed a method for assessing and documenting various aspects of behaviour in a limited time and with minimal disturbance to the baby (Graham 1956, Graham et al. 1956). His method included tests of motor activity and strength; responses to auditory, visual, tactile, and painful stimuli; and measures of irritability and tension.

Based on Graham's early work, Brazelton's (1973) more quantitative scheme relied on 27 items of behaviour and 20 reflex items. In Brazelton's own words, the scale was designed to score the babies' behavioural repertoire and use of states to manage their responsiveness. Such behaviour depends partly, but not only, on factors affecting the infant's neurological state. The examination has often been used as a neurological evaluation. However, it is not suitable for this purpose, as it is a much more global and thus a less specific test to assess neurological integrity. In the early stages, it was compared for its predictive value with other neurological tests. While it gave better predictions of neurological outcome than neurological examinations that were not specifically geared to neonates, this was not the case when it was compared with examinations such as that of Prechtl (Leijon and Finnstrom 1982).

Brazelton's examination was primarily designed as a research tool. It is most valuable when used repeatedly in the neonatal period: the infant serves as her/his own control. Used in this way, the examination can show the process of recovery after events in the perinatal period, such as growth retardation and drug use (Als et al. 1976). It may show differences in responses to such diverse factors as noxious stimuli in the neonatal unit, attitudes of different caregivers, or ethnic influences (Brazelton et al. 1977). Recording these changes in the neonatal period also made it possible to study their effects on later mother–infant interaction. The scale's scope as a research tool was thus very wide. The original test, which was already fairly long, was designed for term infants. The test that was developed later for preterm

3

infants is even longer; therefore, to try to use these tests routinely is patently impractical. Nevertheless, the Brazelton test has made a tremendous impact on the general approach and examination processes in the neonatal unit. It made clinicians aware of the interactive and emotional capabilities of very young infants. Many of the concepts have been incorporated in the evaluation of neonates and have also brought about change in the routine practices of neonatal intensive care units, so that the development of the interactive processes of the newborn infant are interfered with as little as possible. The third edition of the examination (Brazelton and Nugent 1995) added items intended to better elucidate the qualities of the responses of fragile preterm and high-risk infants. Its authors stressed some of the important methodological issues relating to the cultural and ethnic differences in neonatal behaviour, highlighting the variability of behaviour in different settings.

A new approach to neurological assessment, based on the observation of spontaneous motility, has recently been proposed by Prechtl and his collaborators (Prechtl et al. 1997; Cioni et al. 1997). They suggested that the observation of general movements, which are gross movements involving the whole body, is more reliable than the assessment of the incidence of specific isolated movements. General movements, because of their complexity and variability, can be an appropriate indicator of the infant's neurological status. In their studies on low-risk and high-risk preterm and term infants, those authors described the maturation of the normal patterns of general movements in the low-risk infants and the absence of their normal variability and "elegance" in infants with brain lesions. More recently, those authors also showed that the assessment of general movements in the neonatal period can predict outcome in infants at risk (Cioni et al. 1997). Although this method is quick and relatively easy to perform, the examiners must be trained to interpret the results, and video equipment is needed. As the same authors suggest, the method is a useful extension of traditional protocols of neurological examination but is not meant to replace them.

During the 1960s, we used the Prechtl, Saint-Anne Dargassies, and Brazelton schemes, initially in their original format and subsequently modified to meet our particular needs and circumstances in the assessment of preterm and term infants, both ill and well, in the neonatal unit and also the neonatal intensive care unit. Finding none of them fully satisfactory as a practical tool in the day-to-day assessment of infants, we eventually adopted a different approach to the neurological examination, described in the first edition of this manual (Dubowitz and Dubowitz 1981). During the past 15 years, with continuous use of the examination and cumulative experience with it, we felt the need for modification. The present edition includes an update of the examination and our experience with it.

2
EVOLUTION OF THE PRESENT NEUROLOGICAL SCHEME AND ITS APPLICATIONS

From our experience with schemes for neurological assessment of the newborn, we felt that there was a need for a neurological examination that would

- have a simple, objective recording system, so that it was suitable for staff with no particular expertise or experience in neonatal neurology;
- be applicable to both preterm and term infants;
- be reliable soon after birth, in order to document the influence of drugs, hypoxia, trauma, and other environmental factors in the perinatal period and to identify and prevent or lessen complications;
- take not longer than 15 minutes to carry out and record, so that it could be used as a component of the routine clinical assessment of newborn infants;
- be suitable for repeated examinations of infants, making it possible to document the normal evolution of neurological behaviour in the preterm infant after birth, to compare preterm infants with newborn infants of corresponding postmenstrual age, and to detect deviations in neurological signs and their subsequent evolution.

Choice of items
To achieve our aims, we needed items that would

- be applicable to term infants within 3 days of birth;
- be applicable to preterm infants in an incubator in the first few days of life, and also be suitable for sequential examination of the preterm infant;
- be easy to define and show good interobserver correlation;
- cover aspects of higher neurological function;
- provide a means of assessing ill as well as healthy infants.

PHASE 1
In order to see which items from the various examinations used in the past might meet these criteria and be suitable for inclusion, we tested all the available neurological items in a pilot study of some 50 term infants, recording the findings for the examinations as set out by Saint-Anne Dargassies (1977), Prechtl (1977), and Parmelee and Michaelis (1971) in their respective schemes. Naturally, there was a fair degree of overlap of items. We found the Parmelee method of recording, with the aid of illustrative diagrams and an instruction manual, to be the most reproducible, especially when making comparisons between our

own observations and those of less experienced observers, such as resident staff. Therefore, we compiled an examination in which each item was scored with the aid of diagrams. We retained the Parmelee scoring system, classifying responses as "absent", "decreased", "normal", or "increased". In addition to Parmelee's items, we added items from Brazelton's exam that we thought might reflect higher neurological function rather than Brazelton's "interactions", retaining the 9-point scoring system as in the Brazelton manual.

We then produced for our own use a comprehensive manual of instructions for scoring all the items in our protocol. After a number of trials with this scheme, we produced our first proforma (Fig. 2.1), which was then tested over 2 years on a series of more than 500 babies. The sequence of examination was planned so that those assessments requiring the baby to be in a relatively quiet or sleep state were done first, followed by those items not particularly influenced by the baby's state, and finally by those Brazelton items for which the baby needed to be fully awake. For all the infants studied, at the first examination we also assessed gestational age (Dubowitz et al. 1970) (Fig. 2.2).

On this neurological examination, there was good correlation between ratings by pairs of observers examining the baby independently. However, there were still several obvious problems and shortcomings. The examination took too long, and the need to refer constantly to the instruction manual was tiresome. Also, because the method was based on deviations from a norm that had been standardized by earlier authors for term infants only, it lacked a normal standard for preterm infants. Therefore, it was very difficult to classify a particular response objectively as decreased, normal, or increased for a 32-week, 34-week, or 36-week preterm infant. Some changes in approach were essential if our initial criteria were to be met.

PHASE 2
Because eliminating any of the items already selected for the examination might have reduced its efficiency and sensitivity, we tried to shorten the time needed by streamlining the method of recording and documentation.

We had found that the fastest, most accurate way of assessing and recording the gestational age was to use for each infant a single, flat page containing the charts for superficial and neurological criteria, and to encircle the appropriate items directly on the page. In this way, the gestational age could be assessed and recorded within 2 or 3 minutes. This also provided a permanent record for each infant.

Accordingly, for the neurological assessment, we decided to abandon the approach of relating all responses to a norm, and instead to follow the approach used in our scheme for assessing gestational age, namely, grading each item from its minimum to its maximum response, with intermediate stages that could be easily and objectively defined and clearly recognized. We used a 5-point scale, as we had found that this provided a reasonable number of grades to categorize most neurological items objectively. Because we found Brazelton's 9-point scale somewhat cumbersome and difficult to apply, we also modified the Brazelton neurobehavioural criteria to fit a 5-point scale.

Clear instructions for the elicitation of each response were entered directly onto the recording sheet, followed by descriptions of the 5 (or fewer) grades of response and, wherever possible, illustrative diagrams.

NAME			D.O.B./TIME	
HOSP.	NO.		DATE OF EXAM	
RACE	SEX		AGE	

WEIGHT		E.D.D L.N.M.P.	E.D.D Ult.	
HEIGHT		GESTATIONAL ASSESSMENT	SCORE	WEEKS
HEAD CIRC.				

STATE BEFORE EXAMINATION

			STATE	CRY
		SCORE	REMARKS	a
BRAZELTON	Habituation to light (1,2,3)			
	Habituation to sound (1,2,3)	Rattle:		
		Bell:		
	Response to pinprick (1,2,3)			

BRAZELTON II	SCORE	REMARKS
Defensive movement (4)		
Orientation visual (4)		
Orientation auditory (4,5)		
Alertness (4)		
Consolability (6—5,4,3,2)		
Peak of excitement		
Rapidity of build-up (1,2—6)		
Irritability (3,4,5)		
Tremulousness (all)		
Startles (3-6)		

PARMELEE — STATE AFTER UNDRESSING

SECTION I						STATE	
	ABSENT	DECREASED	NORMAL	INCREASED	ASYM.	b	
TONE Trunk flexion attitude •	A	D	N	I			
Head control (traction) •	A	D	N	I			
Flexion/Neck extension	A	D	N	I			
Extension/Neck flexion	A	D	N	I			
LIMBS Recoil arm	L R	L R	L R	L R			
Traction arm	L R	L R	L R	L R			
Recoil leg	L R	L R	L R	L R			
Traction leg	L R	L R	L R	L R			
Ventral suspension •	L R	L R	L R	L R			
MOVEMENT						c	
Head raising, prone	A	D	N	I			
Arm release, prone	A	D	N	I			
PRIMITIVE REFLEXES						d	
Galant	L R	L R	L R	L R		e	
Sucking	A	D	N	I			
Rooting	L R	L R	L R	L R			
Palmar grasp •	L R	L R	L R	L R			
Startle	A	D	N	I			
Leg withdraw	A	D	N	I			
Moro	L R	L R	L R	L R		f	
WALKING REFLEX •	A	D	N	I			
PARMELEE RAW SCORE							
PARMELEE CORRECTED SCORE							

PARMELEE SECTION II					
Cry	Absent	Normal	Excessive	Pitch	Rhythmic	Grunt
Abnormal eye movements	None	Present (describe)			
Tremors	None	Present			
Body movements	Normal	Abnormal (describe)			
Facial weakness	None	Present			

ST. ANNE DARGASSIES ABNORMAL INVENTORY:

Sensory	Alertness	Motility	Cry
Tone of body axis	Ocular signs	SCORE:	

REMARKS:

Note: Do not include in Parmelee score items marked •

Pethidine   Epidural   Other

Fig. 2.1. Prototype proforma for the neurological examination of the newborn infant (1970s).

7

GESTATIONAL AGE CHART

(Dubowitz Score)

Name _____

Hospital No. _____

Sex _____ Race _____

Date/time of birth _____

Date/time of examination _____

Age _____

Weight _____

Length _____

Head circumference _____

Score   Neurological _____

Superficial _____

Total _____

FDD (certain/uncertain) _____

Gest by dates _____

Gest by Assessment _____

Comments _____

Neurological Criteria

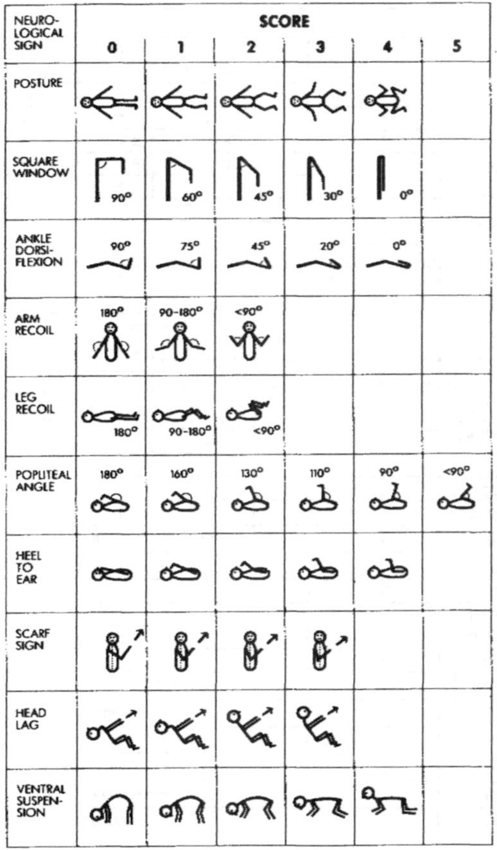

NEUROLOGICAL SIGN	SCORE 0	1	2	3	4	5
POSTURE						
SQUARE WINDOW	90°	60°	45°	30°	0°	
ANKLE DORSIFLEXION	90°	75°	45°	20°	0°	
ARM RECOIL	180°	90–180°	<90°			
LEG RECOIL	180°	90–180°	<90°			
POPLITEAL ANGLE	180°	160°	130°	110°	90°	<90°
HEEL TO EAR						
SCARF SIGN						
HEAD LAG						
VENTRAL SUSPENSION						

External (superficial) Criteria

EXTERNAL SIGN	SCORE 0	1	2	3	4
OEDEMA	Obvious oedema hands and feet; pitting over tibia	No obvious oedema hands and feet; pitting over tibia	No oedema		
SKIN TEXTURE	Very thin, gelatinous	Thin and smooth	Smooth; medium thickness. Rash or superficial peeling	Slight thickening. Superficial cracking and peeling esp. hands and feet	Thick and parchment-like; superficial or deep cracking
SKIN COLOUR (infant not crying)	Dark red	Uniformly pink	Pale pink; variable over body	Pale. Only pink over ears, lips, palms or soles	
SKIN OPACITY (trunk)	Numerous veins and venules clearly seen, especially over abdomen	Veins and tributaries seen	A few large vessels clearly seen over abdomen	A few large vessels seen indistinctly over abdomen	No blood vessels seen
LANUGO (over back)	No lanugo	Abundant, long and thick over whole back	Hair thinning especially over lower back	Small amount of lanugo and bald areas	At least half of back devoid of lanugo
PLANTAR CREASES	No skin creases	Faint red marks over anterior half of sole	Definite red mark over more than anterior half; indentations over less than anterior third	Indentations over more than anterior third	Definite deep indentations over more than anterior third
NIPPLE FORMATION	Nipple barely visible; no areola	Nipple well defined; areola smooth and flat, diameter <0.75 cm	Areola stippled, edge not raised, diameter <0.75 cm	Areola stippled, edge raised, diameter >0.75 cm	
BREAST SIZE	No breast tissue palpable	Breast tissue on one or both sides <0.5 cm diameter	Breast tissue both sides; one or both 0.5–1.0 cm	Breast tissue both sides; one or both >1 cm	
EAR FORM	Pinna flat and shapeless, little or no incurving of edge	Incurving of part of edge of pinna	Partial incurving whole of upper pinna	Well-defined incurving whole of upper pinna	
EAR FIRMNESS	Pinna soft, easily folded, no recoil	Pinna soft, easily folded, slow recoil	Cartilage to edge of pinna, but soft in places, ready recoil	Pinna firm, cartilage to edge; instant recoil	
GENITALIA MALE	Neither testis in scrotum	At least one testis high in scrotum	At least one testis right down		
FEMALES (with hips abducted)	Labia majora widely separated, labia minora protruding	Labia majora almost cover labia minora	Labia majora completely cover labia minora		

(Adapted from Farr et al Develop. Med. Child Neurol. 1966, 8, 507)

Fig. 2.2. Gestational age chart (Dubowitz et al. 1970).

This approach proved to be immensely practical and easy to handle, in spite of the large number of items used, and we soon found that it would meet the various requirements we had initially outlined. In the light of our subsequent experience, we have modified the method in various ways. Some items have been deleted. These include, for example, auditory orientation to a bell, which seemed an unnecessary duplication of a similar response to a rattle, despite the different pitches of the two stimuli. The assessment of withdrawal from a pinprick often upset the mother (whom we always encouraged to observe the examination if she wished) and in any event did not prove to be particularly discriminative in pathological conditions. We also eliminated the test for Galant's (spinal incurvation) reflex, which seemed to be present in all the infants studied. On the other hand, some items that had been excluded were later reintroduced. We noticed that the popliteal angle in certain preterm infants was strikingly at odds with their general state of limb tone and that some infants' degree of head lag when they were pulled from a supine position to a sitting position seemed to be at odds with their head control when they were suspended in a ventral position. Therefore, we thought these two signs (which already formed part of our gestational assessment) might have additional discriminative value relating to the neurological well-being of the infant, apart from reflecting the maturation of the nervous system with increasing gestational age. The items on tendon reflexes, which we had removed from the examination early on when they seemed to be of little discriminative value, were restored when we noticed that residents had taken their removal as a cue to relieve them of the responsibility for eliciting tendon jerks in their routine clinical examination of newborn infants, even in overtly pathological circumstances such as when infants were floppy, hypertonic, or paralysed.

In order to keep the system flexible, we have tried to establish a means of documenting the neurological status of the infant that would be practical for repeated use with the same infant during its maturation from a preterm to a term state, and also with the ill infant. We achieved this by avoiding the use of a single total score, and recording instead a pattern of responses to reflect different aspects of neurological function, thus reducing the need to assess every single item at every examination. The scheme contains enough items on which even a very ill infant can be assessed to give a baseline indication of neurological status for sequential assessment. In addition, items can be added or replaced within the scheme to meet particular requirements in special circumstances or relating to specific studies.

We have not included in the scheme the basic physical examination relevant to the nervous system, such as palpation of sutures and fontanelles and so forth, but assume that this will form part of the general clinical examination of the infant. Our scheme is aimed particularly at recording the functional state of the nervous system.

PHASE 3

Phase 3 was the publication of our methodology in a previous volume of this series (Dubowitz and Dubowitz 1981). The methodology was described in detail and the examination was scored on a proforma (Fig. 2.3; overleaf). This occupied two A4 (297×210 mm) pages and incorporated instructions on the left side of the page, spaces for scoring with the aid of diagrams, and three columns on the right for the recording of the infant's state, asymmetry of response,

NAME.

HOSP. NO.

RACE SEX

D.O.B./TIME

DATE OF EXAM

AGE

WEIGHT

HEIGHT

HEAD CIRC.

E.D.D. L.N.M.P.

E.D.D. U/snd.

GESTATIONAL ASSESSMENT SCORE WEEKS

STATES
1. Deep sleep, no movement, regular breathing.
2. Light sleep, eyes shut, some movement.
3. Dozing, eyes opening and closing.
4. Awake, eyes open, minimal movement.
5. Wide awake, eyes open, vigorous movement.
6. Crying.

HABITUATION (≤ state 3)

Light
Repetitive flashlight stimuli (10) with 5 sec. gap. Shutdown = 2 consecutive negative responses

No response	A. Blink response to first stimulus. B. Tonic blink response. C. Variable response.	A. Shutdown of movement but blink persists 2-5 stimuli. B. Complete shutdown 2-5 stimuli.	A. Shutdown of movement but blink persists 6-10 stimuli. B. Complete shutdown 6-10 stimuli.	A. Equal response to 10 stimuli. B. Infant comes to fully alert state. C. Startles + major responses throughout.

Rattle
Repetitive stimuli (10) with 5 sec gap.

No response	A. Slight movement to first stimulus. B. Variable response.	Startle or movement 2-5 stimuli, then shutdown	Startle or movement 6-10 stimuli, then shutdown	A. B. Grading as above C.

MOVEMENT & TONE

Undress infant

Posture
(At rest - predominant) *

	(hips abducted)	(hips abducted)	(hips adducted)	Abnormal postures: A. Opisthotonus. B. Unusual leg extension. C. Asym. tonic neck reflex

Arm Recoil
Infant supine. Take both hands, extend parallel to the body; hold approx. 2 secs. and release.

No flexion within 5 sec. R L	Partial flexion at elbow >100° within 4-5 sec. R L	Arms flex at elbow to <100° within 2-3 sec. R L	Sudden jerky flexion at elbow immediately after release to ≤60° R L	Difficult to extend; arm snaps back forcefully

Arm Traction
Infant supine; head midline; grasp wrist, slowly pull arm to vertical. Angle of arm scored and resistance noted at moment infant is initially lifted off mattress. Do other arm.

Arm remains fully extended R L	Weak flexion maintained only momentarily R L	Arm flexed at elbow to <140° and maintained 5 sec. R L	Arm flexed at approx. 100° and maintained R L	Strong flexion of arm <100° and maintained R L

Leg Recoil
First flex hips for 5 secs, then extend both legs of infant by traction on ankles; hold down on the bed for 2 secs and release.

No flexion within 5 sec.	Incomplete flexion of hips within 5 sec.	Complete flexion within 5 sec.	Instantaneous complete flexion	Legs cannot be extended; snap back forcefully

Leg Traction
Infant supine. Grasp leg near ankle and slowly pull toward vertical until buttocks 1-2" off. Note resistance at knee and score angle. Do other leg.

No flexion R L	Partial flexion, rapidly lost R L	Knee flexion 140-160° and maintained R L	Knee flexion 100-140° and maintained R L	Strong resistance; flexion <100° R L

Test					
Popliteal angle Infant supine. Approximate knee and thigh to abdomen; extend leg by gentle pressure with index finger behind ankle.	180-160° R L	150-140° R L	130-120° R L	110-90° R L	<90° R L
Head control (post.neck muscles) Grasp infant by shoulders and raise to sitting position; allow head to fall forward; wait 30 sec.	No attempt to raise head	Unsuccessful attempt to raise head upright	Head raised smoothly to upright in 30 sec. but not maintained.	Head raised smoothly to upright in 30 sec. and maintained	Head cannot be flexed forward
Head control (ant.neck muscles) Allow head to fall backward as you hold shoulders; wait 30 sec.	Grading as above	Grading as above	Grading as above	Grading as above	
Head lag * Pull infant toward sitting posture by traction on both wrists. Also note arm flexion.					
Ventral suspension * Hold infant in ventral suspension; observe curvature of back, flexion of limbs and relation of head to trunk.					
Head raising in prone position Infant in prone position with head in midline.	No response	Rolls head to one side	Weak effort to raise head and turns raised head to one side	Infant lifts head, nose and chin off	Strong prolonged head lifting
Arm release in prone position Head in midline. Infant in prone position; arms extended alongside body with palms up.	No effort	Some effort and wriggling	Flexion effort but neither wrist brought to nipple level	One or both wrists brought at least to nipple level without excessive body movement	Strong body movement with both wrists brought to face or 'press-ups'
Spontaneous body movement during examination (supine) If no spont.movement try to elicit by cutaneous stim.	None or minimal	A.Sluggish. B.Random, incoordinated. C.Mainly stretching.	Smooth movements alternating with random, stretching, athetoid or jerky	Smooth alternating movements of arms and legs with medium speed and intensity	Mainly: A.Jerky movement. B.Athetoid movement. C.Other abnormal movement.
Tremors Mark: Fast (>6/sec) or Slow (<6/sec)	No tremor	Tremors only in state 5-6	Tremors only in sleep or after Moro and startles	Some tremors in state 4	Tremulousness in all states
Startles	No startles	Startles to sudden noise, Moro, bang on table only	Occasional spontaneous startle	2-5 spontaneous startles	6+ spontaneous startles
Abnormal movement or posture	No abnormal movement	A. Hands clenched but open intermittently. B. Hands do not open with Moro.	A. Some mouthing movement. B. Intermittent adducted thumb	A. Persistently adducted thumb. B. Hands clenched all the time.	A. Continuous mouthing movement. B. Convulsive movements.

Fig. 2.3 continues

11

(*Fig. 2.3, continued*)

REFLEXES

	Absent	Present	Exaggerated	Clonus	State	Comment	Asymmetry
Tendon reflexes Biceps jerk, Knee jerk, Ankle jerk	Absent	Present	Exaggerated	Clonus			
Palmar grasp Head in midline. Put index finger from ulnar side into hand and gently press palmar surface. Never touch dorsal side of hand.	Absent	Short, weak flexion	Medium strength and sustained flexion for several secs.	Strong flexion; contraction spreads to forearm	Very strong; infant easily lifts off couch		
Rooting Infant supine, head midline. Touch each corner of the mouth in turn (stroke laterally).	No response	A. Partial weak head turn but no mouth opening. B. Mouth opening, no head turn.	Mouth opening on stimulated side with partial head turning	Full head turning, with or without mouth opening	Mouth opening with very jerky head turning		
Sucking Infant supine; place index finger (pad towards palate) in infant's mouth; Judge power of sucking movement after 5 sec.	No attempt	Weak sucking movement: A. Regular. B. Irregular.	Strong sucking movement, poor stripping: A. Regular. B. Irregular.	Strong regular sucking movement with continuing sequence of 5 movements. Good stripping.	Clenching but no regular sucking.		
Walking (state 4,5) Hold infant upright, feet touching bed, neck held straight with fingers.	Absent	Some effort but not continuous with both legs	At least 2 steps with both legs	A. Stork posture; no movement. B. Automatic walking.			
Moro One hand supports infant's head in midline, the other the back. Raise infant to 45° and when infant is relaxed let his head fall through 10°. Note if jerky. Repeat 3 times.	No response, or opening of hands only	Full abduction at the shoulder and extension of the arm	Full abduction but only delayed or partial adduction	Partial abduction at shoulder and extension of arms followed by smooth adduction. A. Abd>Add B. Abd=Add C. Abd>Add	A. No abduction or adduction; extension only. B. Marked adduction only.		

NEUROBEHAVIOURAL ITEMS

					State	Comment	Asymmetry
EYE APPEARANCES	Sunset sign Nerve palsy	Transient nystagmus. Strabismus. Some roving eye movement	Does not open eyes	Normal conjugate eye movement	A. Persistent nystagmus. B. Frequent roving movement. C. Frequent rapid blinks.		
AUDITORY ORIENTATION (state 3,4) To rattle. (Note presence of startle.)	A. No reaction. B. Auditory startle but no true orientation.	Brightens and stills; may turn toward stimuli with eyes closed	Alerting and shifting of eyes; head may or may not turn to source	Alerting; prolonged head turns to stimulus; search with eyes	Turning and alerting to stimulus each time on both sides		

	Does not focus or follow stimulus	Stills; focuses on stimulus; may follow 30° jerkily; does not find stimulus again spontaneously	Follows 30-60° horizontally; may follow vertically; does not lose stimulus but finds it again. Brief vertical glance	Follows with eyes and head horizontally and to some extent vertically, with frowning	Sustained fixation; follows vertically, horizontally, and in circle
VISUAL ORIENTATION (state 4) To red woollen ball					
ALERTNESS (state 4)	Inattentive; rarely or never responds to direct stimulation	When alert, periods rather brief; rather variable response to orientation	When alert, alertness moderately sustained; may use stimulus to come to alert state	Sustained alertness; orientation frequent, reliable to visual but not auditory stimuli	Continuous alertness, which does not seem to tire, to both auditory and visual stimuli
DEFENSIVE REACTION A cloth or hand is placed over the infant's face to partially occlude the nasal airway.	No response	A. General quietening. B. Non-specific activity with long latency.	Rooting; lateral neck turning; possibly neck stretching	Swipes with arm	Swipes with arm with rather violent body movement
PEAK OF EXCITEMENT	Low level arousal to all stimuli; never > state 3	Infant reaches state 4-5 briefly but predominantly in lower states	Infant predominantly state 4 or 5; may reach state 6 after stimulation but returns to lower state spontaneously	Infant reaches state 6 but can be consoled relatively easily	A. Mainly state 6. Difficult to console, if at all. B. Mainly state 4-5 but if reaches state 6 cannot be consoled.
IRRITABILITY (states 3,4,5) Aversive stimuli: Uncover Ventral susp. Undress Moro Pull to sit Walking reflex Prone	No irritable crying to any of the stimuli	Cries to 1-2 stimuli	Cries to 3-4 stimuli	Cries to 5-6 stimuli	Cries to all stimuli
CONSOLABILITY (state 6)	Never above state 5 during examination, therefore not needed	Consoling not needed. Consoles spontaneously	Consoled by talking, hand on belly or wrapping up	Consoled by picking up and holding; may need finger in mouth	Not consolable
CRY	No cry at all	Only whimpering cry	Cries to stimuli but normal pitch	Lusty cry to offensive stimuli; normal pitch	High-pitched cry, often continuous

Record time after feed:

Examiner:

NOTES * If asymmetrical or atypical, draw in on nearest figure

Record any abnormal signs (e.g. facial palsy, contractures, etc.). Draw if possible.

Fig. 2.3. Definitive proforma for the neurological examination of the newborn infant (Dubowitz and Dubowitz 1981).

13

TABLE 2.1
Items included in 1981 protocol for assessing functional state of infant's nervous system (Dubowitz and Dubowitz 1981)

Habituation	Movement and tone	Reflexes	Neurobehaviour	Other
Light	Posture	Tendon	Auditory orientation	Eye appearance
Sound	Arm recoil	Palmar grasp	Visual orientation	Cry
	Arm traction	Rooting	Alertness	
	Leg recoil	Sucking	Defensive reaction	
	Leg traction	Walking	Peak of excitement	
	Popliteal angle	Moro	Irritability	
	Head control		Consolability	
	Posterior neck muscles			
	Anterior neck muscles			
	Head lag			
	Ventral suspension			
	Head raising in prone			
	Arm release in prone			
	Spontaneous body movements			
	Tremors/startles			
	Abnormal movements			

and any additional comment. The items included in the protocol, and their grouping, are shown in Table 2.1.

The behavioural state, which was to be scored next to each item, was graded in six grades, as in Brazelton's scale, and not five as in Prechtl and Beintema's (Table 2.2), since we found that Brazelton's state 3 (drowsy or semi-dozing, with eyes opening and closing), though a transitional state between state 2 and state 4, was frequently present in both preterm and term infants.

PHASE 4

The examination published in 1981 has been in use for 15 years. Although the basic scheme proved to be very successful, in particular in relating lesions to neurological patterns and documenting longitudinal neurological impairment and recovery, it had certain shortcomings. On some items, responses were difficult to elicit, while others, though responses were easily elicited, proved to be relatively superfluous. We also found that some items not originally included could be useful. The scheme has therefore been revised as summarized below.

Items eliminated
The following items were eliminated: *habituation to light and rattle, arm release in the prone, walking reflex, rooting reflex, defensive reaction,* and *peak of excitement*.

- *Habituation to light and sound* was eliminated from the routine proforma because the responses are difficult to elicit routinely in the environment of the neonatal intensive care unit, which is generally noisy and brightly lit. We did, however, retain the description of this item, so that it can be optional for people who want to use it in a specific study, e.g., of the effects of drugs or anaesthetic on the nervous system.

TABLE 2.2
Grading of infant's state

Prechtl and Beintema (1964)

State 1	Eyes closed, regular respiration, no movements
State 2	Eyes closed, irregular respiration, no gross movements
State 3	Eyes open, no gross movements
State 4	Eyes open, gross movements, no crying
State 5	Eyes open or closed, crying

Brazelton (1973)

State 1	Deep sleep with regular breathing, eyes closed, no spontaneous activity, no eye movements
State 2	Light sleep with eyes closed; rapid eye movements, irregular respiration
State 3	Drowsy or semi-dozing; eyes open or closed, activity variable, movements usually smooth
State 4	Alert, with bright look; minimal motor activity
State 5	Eyes open, considerable motor activity
State 6	Crying

- *Arm release in the prone* and *walking reflex* were eliminated because we had not found that they discriminated between normal and abnormal infants.

- *Rooting reflex* was eliminated because the presence of a nasogastric tube often interfered with the reflex.

- *Defensive reaction* was discontinued because the item gave only limited information and many parents found the procedure of covering the infant's face objectionable.

- *Peak of excitement* was eliminated as an individual item but was combined with irritability.

Modifications in items retained

We have redefined the recording of *arm traction, arm recoil,* and *leg recoil* so that the most predominant response can be scored.

- The scoring of *popliteal angle* has been slightly changed, to more easily definable grades.

- *Movements* has been completely redefined in the light of recent work by Prechtl's group. The quality and the quantity of the movements are now scored as two separate items.

- The old item *abnormal movement and posture* has been subdivided, with the movement component incorporated with the movement section and the abnormal posture of hand and foot described separately.

- *Irritability* and *peak of excitement* have been incorporated into one item.

- The item *sucking* has been redefined and now also incorporates the gag response.

- A few minor changes have been made in some of the other items.

New items

We introduced five new items to evaluate the relative distribution of tone, in an attempt to identify normal and abnormal tone patterns. In our experience, abnormal patterns of tone

15

TABLE 2.3
Items included in 1998 protocol for assessing functional state of infant's nervous system

Posture and tone	Tone patterns	Reflexes	Movements	Abnormal signs	Behaviour
Posture	Flexor tone 1	Tendon reflexes	Spontaneous:	Abnormal hand	Eye appearance
Arm recoil	(in supine)	Palmar grasp	Quality	and toe posture	Auditory orientation
Arm traction	Flexor tone 2	Plantar grasp	Quantity	Tremors	Visual orientation
Leg recoil	(arms vs legs)	Sucking reflex	Head raising,	Startles	Alertness
Leg traction	Leg extensor tone	Placing	prone		Irritability
Popliteal angle	Neck extensor tone	Moro response			Consolability
Head control 1	Increased extensor				Cry
(flexor tone)	tone				
Head control 2					
(extensor tone)					
Head lag					
Ventral suspension					

are more often associated with neurological abnormalities than is either generally increased or generally decreased tone.

Other changes
Following these changes, the proforma was restructured in six sections (Table 2.3).

Although the total number of items has not increased, we have spread the proforma (Fig. 2.4) onto three pages in order to increase the font size, because many people, particularly in the Third World, where English is not the first language, found it difficult to cope with the small print (which becomes even less legible on photocopied forms).

The present manual also includes a new chapter describing an optimality score for term infants, for use mainly in a research setting to provide quantification of the neurological examination.

We have also extended the chapter on preterm infants, providing more detailed information on the evolution of neurological signs and their relation to gestational age.

In the light of our experience over the past 15 years with the proforma in parallel with the advent of brain imaging techniques, we have replaced the individual case histories with a more general chapter relating the clinical patterns of neurological abnormalities to a number of brain lesions identified by brain imaging.

Our final chapter describes a number of adaptations of the scheme for selected circumstances. These include a specially adapted version for the assessment of term infants in developing countries by relatively untrained staff; an abbreviated proforma for screening in the postnatal ward; and an adaptation for infants after the neonatal period.

Fig. 2.4 a,b,c *(facing page and overleaf)*. Revised version of the proforma (Dubowitz et al. 1998).

NAME _____ SEX___ RACE_____ D.O.B._____ AGE_____ G.A._____ BW _____

Posture and tone

POSTURE Infant supine. Look mainly at position of legs but also note arms. *Score predominant posture.*	arms & legs extended or very slightly flexed	Legs slightly flexed	legs well flexed but not adducted	legs well flexed & adducted near abdomen	abnormal posture: a) opisthotonus b) marked leg extension, strong arm flexion		
ARM RECOIL Take both hands, quickly extend arms parallel to the body, Count to three. Release. Repeat 3 times.	arms do not flex	arms flex slowly, not always; not completely	arms flex slowly; more completely	arms flex quickly and completely	arms difficult to extend; snap back forcefully		
ARM TRACTION Hold wrist and pull arm upwards. Note flexion at elbow and resistance while shoulder lifts off table. *Test each side separately.*	arms remain straight; no resistance felt	arms flex slightly or some resistance felt	arms flex well till shoulder lifts, then straighten	arms flex at approx 100° & maintained as shoulder lifts	flexion of arms <100°; maintained when body lifts up		
R	L	R	L	R	L	R	L
LEG RECOIL Take *both* ankles in one hand, flex hips + knees. Quickly extend. Release. Repeat 3 times.	No flexion	incomplete or variable flexion	complete but slow flexion	complete fast flexion	legs difficult to extend; snap back forcefully		
LEG TRACTION Grasp ankle and slowly pull leg upwards. Note flexion at knees and resistance as buttocks lift. *Test each side separately.*	legs straight - no resistance felt	legs flex slightly or some resistance felt	legs flex well till bottom lifts up	knee flexes remains flexed when bottom up	flexion stays when back+bottom up		
R	L	R	L	R	L	R	L
POPLITEAL ANGLE Fix knee on abdomen, extend leg by gentle pressure with index finger behind the ankle. Note angle at knee. *Test each side separately.*	180°	≈150°	≈110°	≈00°	<90°		
R	L	R	L	R	L	R	L
HEAD CONTROL (1) *(extensor tone)* Infant sitting upright. Encircle chest with both hands holding shoulders. Let head drop forward.	no attempt to raise head	infant tries: effort better felt than seen	raises head but drops forward or back	raises head: remains vertical; it may wobble			
HEAD CONTROL (2) *(flexor tone)* Infant sitting upright. Encircle chest with both hands holding shoulders. Let head drop backward.	no attempt to raise head	infant tries: effort better felt than seen	raises head but drops forward or back	raises head: remains vertical; it may wobble	head upright or extended; cannot be passively flexed		
HEAD LAG Pull infant towards sitting posture by traction on both wrists & support head slightly. Also note arm flexion.	head drops & stays back	tries to lift head but it drops back	able to lift head slightly	lifts head in line with body	head in front of body		
VENTRAL SUSPENSION Hold infant in ventral suspension. Observe back, flexion of limbs, and relation of head to trunk. If it looks different, DRAW.	back curved, head & limbs hang straight	back curved, head ↓, limbs slightly flexed	back slightly curved, limbs flexed	back straight, head in line, limbs flexed	back straight, head above body		

Fig. 2.4a.

17

Tone patterns

FLEXOR TONE (1) **(on traction: arm versus leg)** Compare scores of arm traction with leg traction.		score for arm flexion less than leg flexion	score for arm flexion equal to leg flexion	score for arm flexion more than leg flexion but difference 1 column or less	score for arm flexion more than leg flexion but difference more than 1 column		
FLEXOR TONE (2) **(arm versus leg)** Posture in supine.			arms and legs flexed	strong arm flexion with strong leg extension *intermittent*	strong arm flexion with strong leg extension *continuous*		
LEG EXTENSOR TONE Compare scores of leg traction and popliteal angle.		score for leg traction more than score for popliteal angle	score for leg traction equal to score for popliteal angle	score for leg traction less than score for popliteal angle, by 1 column only	score for leg traction less than score for popliteal angle, by more than 1 column		
NECK EXTENSOR TONE (SITTING) Compare scores of head control 1 and 2.		score for head extension less than head flexion	score for head extension equal to head flexion	score for head extension more than head flexion. but difference 1 column or less	score for head extension more than head flexion but difference more than 1 column		
INCREASED EXTENSOR TONE (HORIZONTAL) Compare scores of head lag and ventral suspension.		score for ventral suspension less than head lag	score for ventral suspension equal to head lag	score for ventral suspension more than head lag but difference 1 column or less	score for ventral suspension more than head lag but difference more than 1 column		

Reflexes

TENDON REFLEX Test biceps, knee, and ankle jerks.	absent	felt, not seen	seen	"exaggerated" (very brisk)	clonus		
SUCK / GAG Little finger into mouth with pulp of finger upwards.	no gag / no suck	weak irregular suck only No stripping	weak regular suck Some stripping	strong suck: (a) irregular (b) regular Good stripping	no suck but strong clenching		
PALMAR GRASP Put index finger into the hand and gently press palmar surface. Do not touch dorsal surface. *Test each side separately.*	no response R L	short, weak flexion of fingers R L	strong flexion of fingers R L	strong finger flexion, shoulder ↑ R L	very strong grasp; infant can be lifted off couch R L		
PLANTAR GRASP Press thumb on the sole below the toes. *Test each side separately.*	no response R L	partial plantar flexion of toes R L	toes curve around the examiner's finger R L				
PLACING Lift infant in an upright position and stroke the dorsum of the foot against a protruding edge of a flat surface. *Test each side separately.*	no response R L	dorsiflexion of ankle only R L	full placing response with flexion of hip and knee & placing sole on surface R L				
MORO REFLEX One hand supports infant's head in midline, the other the back. Raise infant to 45° and when infant is relaxed let head fall through 10°. Note if jerky. Repeat 3 times.	no response, or opening of hands only	full abduction at shoulder and extension of the arms; no adduction 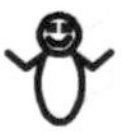	full abduction, but only delayed or partial adduction 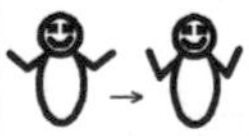	partial abduction at shoulder, and extension of arms followed by smooth adduction 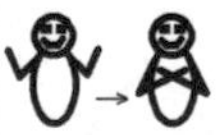	• minimal abduction or adduction • no abduction or adduction; only forward extension of arms • marked adduction only 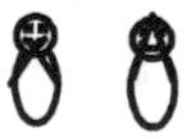		

or

Fig. 2.4b.

18

Movements

SPONTANEOUS MOVEMENT (quantity) Watch infant lying supine.	no movement	sporadic and short isolated movements	frequent isolated movements	frequent generalized movements	continuous exaggerated movements	
SPONTANEOUS MOVEMENT (quality) Watch infant lying supine.	only stretches	stretches and random abrupt movements; some smooth movements	fluent movements but monotonous	fluent alternating movements of arms + legs; good variability	• cramped, synchronized; • mouthing • jerky or other abnormal movements	
HEAD RAISING PRONE Infant in prone, head in midline.	no response	infant rolls head over, chin not raised	infant raises chin, rolls head over	infant brings head and chin up	infant brings head up and keeps it up	

Abnormal signs/patterns

ABNORMAL HAND OR TOE POSTURES		hands open, toes straight most of the time	intermittent fisting or thumb adduction	continuous fisting or thumb adduction; index finger flexion, thumb opposition	continuous big toe extension or flexion of all toes	
TREMOR		no tremor, or tremor only when crying or only after Moro reflex	tremor occasionally when awake	frequent tremors when awake	continuous tremors	
STARTLE	no startle even to sudden noise	no spontaneous startle but reacts to sudden noise	2-3 spontaneous startles	more than 3 spontaneous startles	continuous startles	

Orientation and behaviour

EYE APPEARANCES	does not open eyes		full conjugated eye movements	*transient* • nystagmus • strabismus • roving eye movements • sunset sign	*persistent* • nystagmus • strabismus • roving eye movements abnormal pupils	
AUDITORY ORIENTATION Infant awake. Wrap infant. Hold rattle 10 to 15 cm from ear.	no reaction	auditory startle; brightens and stills; no true orientation	shifting of eyes, head might turn towards source	prolonged head turn to stimulus; search with eyes; smooth	turns head (jerkily, abruptly) & eyes towards noise every time	
VISUAL ORIENTATION Wrap infant, wake up with rattle if needed or rock gently. Note if baby can see and follow red ball (B) or target (T).	does not follow or focus on stimuli	stills, focuses, follows briefly to the side but loses stimuli	follows horizontally and vertically; no head turn	follows horizontally and vertically; turns head	follows in a circle	
			B T	B T	B T	B T
ALERTNESS *Tested as response to visual stimuli* (B or T).	will not respond to stimuli	when awake, looks only briefly	when awake, looks at stimuli but loses them	keeps interest in stimuli	does not tire (hyper-reactive)	
IRRITABILITY In response to stimuli.	quiet all the time, not irritable to any stimuli	awakes, cries sometimes when handled	cries often when handled	cries always when handled	cries even when not handled	
CONSOLABILITY Ease to quiet infant.	not crying; consoling not needed	cries briefly; consoling not needed	cries; becomes quiet when talked to	cries; needs picking up to be consoled	cries; cannot be consoled	
CRY	no cry at all	whimpering cry only	cries to stimuli but normal pitch		High-pitched cry; often continuous	

SUMMARY OF EXAMINATION:

HEAD AND TRUNK TONE: LIMB TONE:

MOTILITY: REFLEXES:

ORIENTATION AND ALERTNESS: IRRITABILITY:

CONSOLABILITY: LIST DEVIANT SIGNS:

Fig. 2.4c.

3
THE NEUROLOGICAL ASSESSMENT

This chapter describes in detail the methodology for our present proforma (see Fig. 2.4).

Timing and sequence of the recording
Many neurological items are influenced by the baby's state, and we have referred earlier to our planning of the sequence of the examination so that items requiring the infant to be sleeping or relatively quiet (states 1 or 2) are elicited first, followed by those not particularly influenced by the state, and finally by the Brazelton behaviour items for which the infant needs to be fully awake (states 4 to 5). We have included an extra column in the proforma to record the state of the infant at the time of assessment of each item.

To ensure that infants are in a comparable state, we try to assess them all about two-thirds of the way between one feed and the next, irrespective of the frequency of the feeds. This usually ensures that the infant is quiet and asleep for the start of the assessment but not too deeply asleep (as it might be too soon after a feed) to become awake and alert enough for the examination to be completed. Also, the time chosen is not so near the time for the next feed that the infant might either already be awake at the start of the examination or be irritable and crying from hunger during the examination. Preterm infants being given continuous feeding (intravenous or alimentary) are examined at any time.

The sequence of items in the proforma is optimal for the infant who is asleep at the beginning of the examination and it ensures that she/he is gradually awoken in the course of the examination. In practice, this order may not always be feasible or optimal: then the of examination can be changed accordingly. If an infant is already fully awake when the examination is started, it is preferable to do the Brazelton orientation items first, as too much initial handling may upset the infant and it may be difficult to get her/him back to an optimal state. In the case of a young preterm infant or an ill infant who can tolerate only minimal handling, one has to be selective about what to do and when. One should do the reflex items, as appropriate, while the infant is in the supine position and then either turn her/him prone for the other items or, if that is not possible, come back for a further examination in the prone or other positions into which the infant may be turned for the sake of clinical management. One has to be guided by the infant's clinical condition and assess only those items that it is practical to do at the time. In infants on ventilators, some items will be impossible to assess, so the examination will be incomplete. In these cases, however, it will still allow at least a sequential comparison to be made on the basis of the items that can be recorded.

In the following section, we define in detail and illustrate the individual neurological criteria retained in the scheme. Unless otherwise stated, each item is graded from 1 (least response) to 5 (most response).

20

Interpretation of individual items

Sometimes it is difficult to decide which definition of a neurological sign is the most appropriate one to circle on the chart. Then it is often easiest to eliminate the obviously inappropriate ones, usually leaving a choice of two. If it is still difficult to decide between these two, and the items are quite different, it may be appropriate to circle both.

For items that are constantly changing, such as posture and type of mobility (Prechtl et al. 1979), we try to record the predominant status during the examination. It rapidly becomes apparent, as with any assessment system, that the newborn infant has not always read the appropriate text and may not be obliging enough to conform exactly to one of the diagrams for a particular response. In such cases, the examiner can circle the figure that most closely resembles the infant's response and record the deviation, be it asymmetry or some other aberration, by drawing it in on the figure. If items are seen to coexist, such as transient nystagmus (Eye appearances, column 4) and conjugate eye movement (column 2), both figures are circled, to record both patterns.

An additional column on the right makes it possible to draw attention to asymmetry of response, which can also be recorded on the diagram itself, since provision has been made throughout the proforma for separate recording of the left and right sides.

We have added a summary to the proforma for recording any specific comments about individual criteria. Any unusual item can be marked with an asterisk and commented on in more detail in the final summary. We tend to use this summary section for observations that cannot readily be fitted into any of the other categories: e.g., poor spontaneous activity but active when stimulated; unusual or aberrant Moro reflex; presence of general illness; or other clinical problems such as cardiac failure, necrotizing enterocolitis, respiratory distress, needing assisted ventilation, and so forth.

Included after the current items in this chapter are some additional ones that were not retained in the present proforma but that can still sometimes be useful.

POSTURE AND TONE

POSTURE

Method

Posture is assessed with the infant supine and the head in the midline, after gently uncovering the infant and taking off or loosening the nappy (diaper), with as little disturbance as possible (Fig. 3.1.).

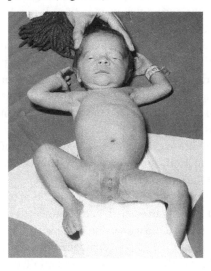

Fig. 3.1.

Scoring posture

arms & legs extended or very slightly flexed	Legs slightly flexed	legs well flexed but not adducted	legs well flexed & adducted near abdomen	abnormal posture: a) opisthotonus b) marked leg extension, strong arm flexion

Because posture changes if the infant is moving, the posture recorded is the predominant one when the infant is in a quiet state. We have defined four grades of posture with increasing flexion of the limbs and have added a fifth grade, unusual or abnormal postures. The diagram most resembling the infant's posture is ringed (Figs. 3.2–3.7).

Cautionary tales

It is important to document the observed posture consistently and accurately. If it does not exactly match any of the diagrams, the diagram most resembling the leg position is circled and is then amended to show the infant's arm position or any asymmetry. The observer can use her/his own discretion so long as the record will be clear and unambiguous when it is referred to later for comparison. Posture is greatly influenced by the infant's state, particularly by crying. If no recording can be made with the infant in a quiet state, this should be noted.

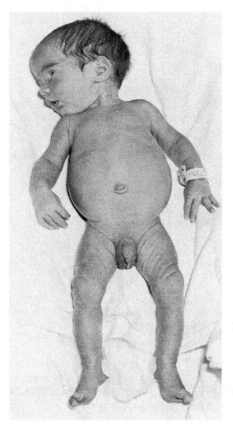

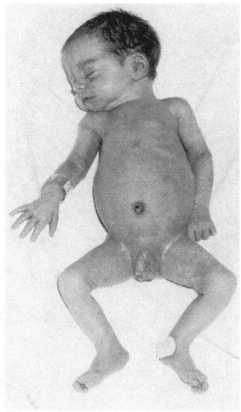

Fig. 3.2. Posture. Slight flexion of legs and of elbows. Score 1. Some infants may show flexion of arms together with partial flexion of legs, appropriate for score 1 or 2; in such cases, it is more reliable to base assessment on posture of legs, and to draw in observed arm position.

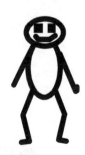

Fig. 3.3. Posture. More marked flexion of legs; slight flexion of arms. Score 2.

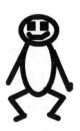

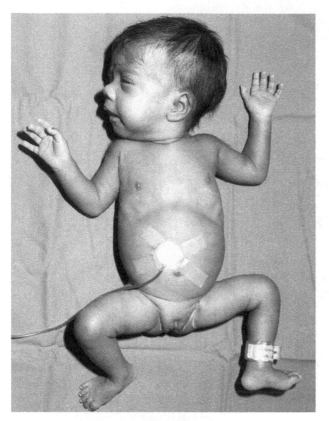

Fig. 3.4. Posture. More marked flexion of legs and arms; hips abducted. Score 3.

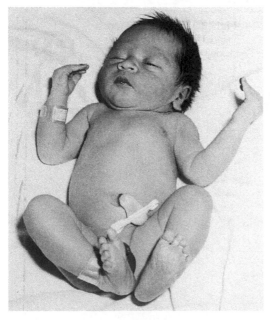

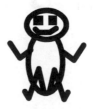

Fig. 3.5. Posture. Full flexion of arms and legs. Hips adducted. Score 4.

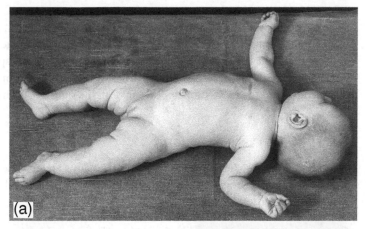

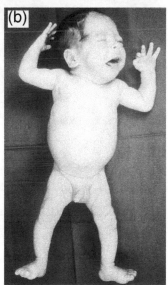

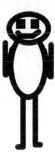

Fig. 3.6. Abnormal postures.
(a) Opisthotonus; (b) marked leg
extension with strong arm flexion.

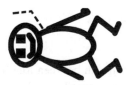

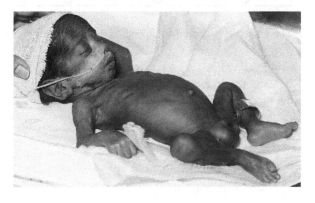

Fig. 3.7. Asymmetrical posture. If
the posture observed does not exactly
coincide with any of the diagrams
on the proforma, the nearest diagram
can be circled and amended as
appropriate.

25

TONE IN THE LIMBS

Tone in the limbs is assessed from arm and leg traction and recoil, and from the popliteal angle. All these assessments are made with the infant in the supine position and the head in the midline (the head can be steadied with a rolled-up nappy [diaper] on either side). All items are scored separately for the two sides, and a difference of one grade or more is recorded by ticking the "asymmetry" column on the right of the chart.

ARM RECOIL

Method

The infant is supine, the head in the midline. The arms are extended by pulling the hands alongside the trunk, holding them for 1 or 2 seconds, and then releasing them (Fig. 3.8). The two arms are tested simultaneously.

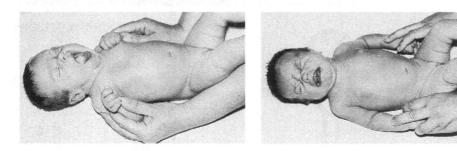

Fig. 3.8. Testing arm recoil.

Scoring arm recoil

1	2	3	4	5
arms do not flex	arms flex slowly, not always; not completely	arms flex slowly; more completely	arms flex quickly and completely	arms difficult to extend; snap back forcefully

The response is scored for speed of recoil and angle at the elbow.

Cautionary tales

In some very premature infants, it can be difficult to distinguish between true recoil and the random movements, sometimes resembling an incomplete recoil, that the manoeuvre often initiates.

ARM TRACTION

Method

The infant is supine, the head in the midline. Each arm is tested separately. The arm is slowly pulled to a vertical position by traction on the wrist (Fig. 3.9).

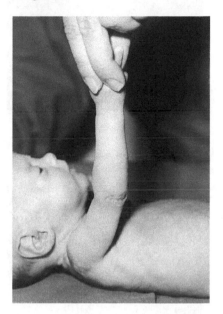

Fig. 3.9. Arm traction test.

Scoring arm traction test

1	2	3	4	5
arms remain straight; no resistance felt	arms flex slightly or some resistance felt	arms flex well till shoulder lifts, then straighten	arms flex at approx 100° & maintained as shoulder lifts	flexion of arms <100°; maintained when body lifts up

The resistance is noted and the angle at the elbow is scored when the infant's shoulder lifts from the surface. In some infants, the response is better felt than seen; in others, flexion is well maintained only until the shoulder is raised. The infant's response is matched to the nearest diagram (Figs. 3.10–3.12).

Cautionary tales

Avoid pulling by the infant's hand, as this produces a palmar grasp response. Some observers differ in their interpretation of the amount of resistance present (especially between grades 2 and 3), but individual observers seem to be consistent in their own scoring. Good interobserver training is therefore essential.

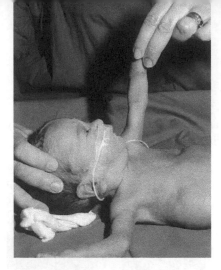

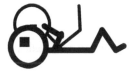

Fig. 3.10. Arm traction test. Arms remain straight, no resistance. Score 1.

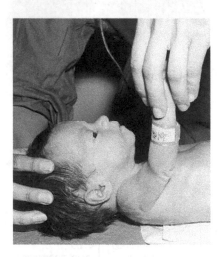

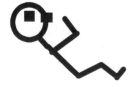

Fig. 3.11. Arm traction test. Good flexion of arms. Flexion is well maintained until shoulder is elevated. Score 3.

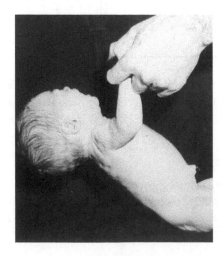

Fig. 3.12. Arm traction test. Full flexion of arms maintained even when body lifts up. Score between 4 and 5,

LEG RECOIL
Method
The two ankles are held in one hand and the legs are fully flexed for about 5 seconds (to ensure the infant is fully relaxed), and then are fully extended and released after 1 or 2 seconds (Fig. 3.13). The test is repeated three times and the predominant response is recorded.

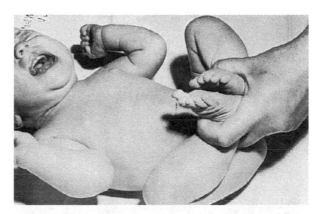

Fig. 3.13. Testing leg recoil.

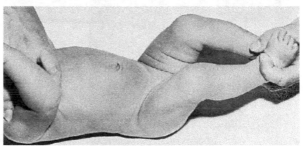

Scoring leg recoil

1	2	3	4	5
No flexion	incomplete or variable flexion	complete but slow flexion	complete fast flexion	legs difficult to extend; snap back forcefully

The response is scored according to the speed and completeness of the recoil, using the predominant reponse.

Cautionary tales
If the infant is actively stretching when the test is done, it is worth repeating the test: in this case, the best response is scored. If the infant is stretching continually and this results in incomplete recoil, that should be noted: in our experience, at times this seems to relate to increased extensor tone.

LEG TRACTION

Method

The infant is supine, the head in the midline. Each leg is tested separately, by raising it into a vertical position using gentle traction on the ankle (Fig. 3.14). The manoeuvre is repeated three times and the predominant response is recorded.

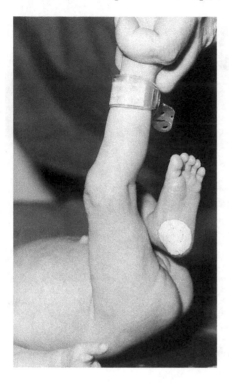

Fig. 3.14. Leg traction test.

Scoring leg traction test

legs straight - no resistance felt	legs flex slightly or some resistance felt	legs flex well till bottom lifts up	knee flexes remains flexed when bottom up	flexion stays when back+bottom up
R L	R L	R L	R L	R L

The resistance and the angle at the knee are noted when the buttock becomes elevated from the surface. The diagram most resembling the response is circled (Figs 3.15–3.17).

Cautionary tales

This response is to some extent state-dependent and the infant should not be tested in state 1 or 6. The response may vary if it is elicited by traction on the foot or higher up on the leg: therefore, consistency in the methodology is important.

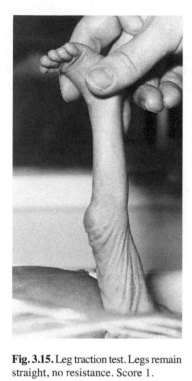

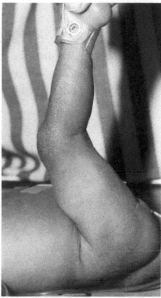

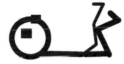

Fig. 3.16. Good flexion of knee (approximately 140°). Flexion is well maintained until body is elevated from surface. Score 3.

Fig. 3.15. Leg traction test. Legs remain straight, no resistance. Score 1.

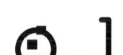

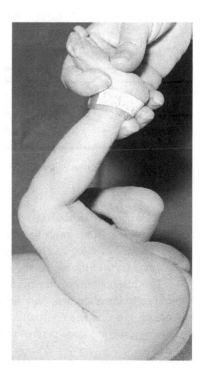

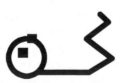

Fig. 3.17. Full flexion of knee maintained even when body lifts up. Score 4.

POPLITEAL ANGLE

Method

The infant is supine, the head in the midline. Each leg is tested separately. The examiner holds the thigh against the infant's abdomen by grasping the knee between thumb and index finger, and then extends the leg by pressing the back of the ankle with the other index finger and stopping when resistance is felt (Fig 3.18).

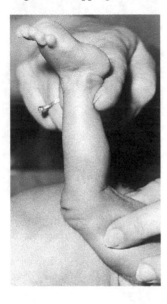

Fig. 3.18. Testing popliteal angle.

Scoring popliteal angle

1	2	3	4	5
180°	≈ 150°	≈110°	≈90°	<90°

The angle of the knee is scored by circling the appropriate diagram (Fig. 3.19–3.22).

Cautionary tales

The angle observed depends on how hard the examiner pushes the leg. One of the most common errors is to record the angle between the lower leg and the examining table rather than that between the lower leg and the thigh (so that, for example, a 110° angle between the upper and lower parts of the leg, as shown in column 3, might be incorrectly recorded as 90°).

This manoeuvre is different from the one described by French authors. Because we hold the knee to the abdomen, only the tightness in the hamstrings is measured. If that is not done, the hip extension will affect the response. Premature infants and some infants with pathological conditions may show very different findings if tested in these two different ways.

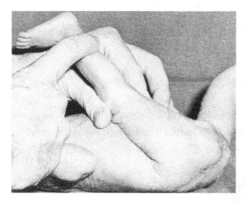

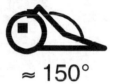

180°

Fig. 3.19. Popliteal angle 180°. Score 1.

Fig. 3.20. Popliteal angle approximately 150°. Score 2.

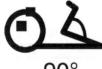

≈ 150°

≈90°

Fig. 3.21. Popliteal angle approximately 90°. Score 4.

Fig. 3.22. Popliteal angle less than 90°. Score 5.

<90°

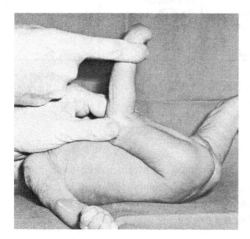

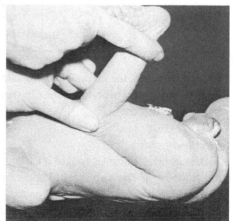

TRUNK AND NECK TONE

Trunk and neck tone are reflected in the items assessing head control, as well as in the posture already observed above.

HEAD CONTROL (1) – POSTERIOR NECK MUSCLES (EXTENSOR TONE)

Method

The infant, in a sitting position, is held by the shoulders, with the examiner's hands encircling the chest. The head is allowed to fall forward. The infant's ability to raise the head to a vertical position within 30 seconds is noted (Fig. 3.23).

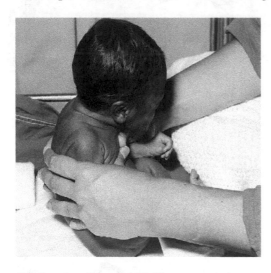

Fig. 3.23. Testing for head control (1) (extensor tone).

Scoring head control (1) (extensor tone)

1	2	3	4	5
no attempt to raise head	infant tries: effort better felt than seen	raises head but drops forward or back	raises head: remains vertical; it may wobble	

In the first grade, the infant's head remains flexed and cannot be brought back; there are three further grades of ability to raise the head into an extended position. A fifth grade shows inability to flex the head.

Cautionary tales

Make sure that the infant is upright. If the infant is leaning back or forward, more effort is required to lift the head. The item is tested and scored differently from a similar item in the French examination. We found that scores on the French method varied widely between observers, particularly inexperienced ones, as the speed of the manoeuvre affects the infant's response.

HEAD CONTROL (2) – ANTERIOR NECK MUSCLES (FLEXOR TONE)
Method
This is similar to the previous item, with the infant in a sitting position and held by the shoulders, but here the head is allowed to extend fully (i.e., to fall back). The degree of head flexion within 30 seconds is noted (Fig. 3.24).

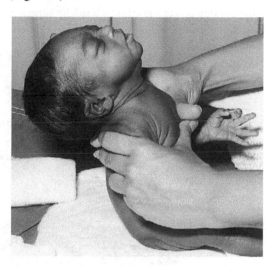

Fig. 3.24. Testing for head control (2) (flexor tone).

Scoring head control (2) (flexor tone)

1	2	3	4	5
no attempt to raise head	infant tries: effort better felt than seen	raises head but drops forward or back	raises head: remains vertical; it may wobble	head upright or extended; cannot be passively flexed

In the first grade (column 1), the infant's head remains extended and is not brought forward at all; the next three diagrams show grades of ability to bring the head into a flexed position.

Cautionary tales
Make sure that the infant is upright. If the infant is leaned back or forward, more effort is required to lift the head. The comments about the French method in the previous item also apply here.

HEAD LAG (RESPONSE TO TRACTION)

Method

With the infant supine, the wrists are grasped together and the infant is gently pulled towards the sitting position. The posture of the head is noted when the shoulders are elevated to about 45° (Fig. 3.25). In premature babies, particularly, the examiner should avoid hyperextension of the infant's head, by supporting it with one hand and pulling up with the other.

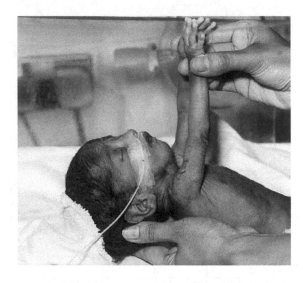

Fig. 3.25. Testing head lag.

Scoring head lag

1	2	3	4	5
head drops & stays back	tries to lift head but it drops back	able to lift head slightly	lifts head in line with body	head in front of body

One of five grades of response is ringed, on the basis of the head position (Figs. 3.26–3.29).

Cautionary tales

If the flexion response in the arms does not correspond to that in the diagrams, the diagram that most closely reflects the head posture should be ringed and the deviation of the arms should be drawn in. It is important to document such deviation, because (for example) some infants, such as those with bronchopulmonary dysplasia, may show marked head lag in association with well-flexed arms. This should alert the examiner to the possibility of increased extensor tone in the neck and trunk muscles, which is usually abnormal. On the other hand, normal preterm infants reaching 40 weeks postmenstrual age may show good head control in association with completely extended arms.

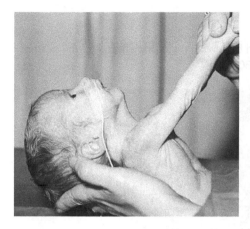
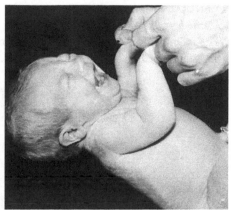

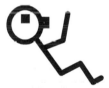

Fig. 3.26. Head lag. Complete head drop. Note relation between ear and shoulder. Score 1.

Fig. 3.27. Head lag. Good attempts to lift the head, but it drops back. Score 2.

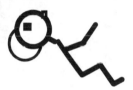

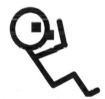

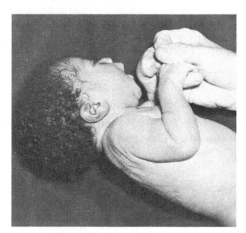
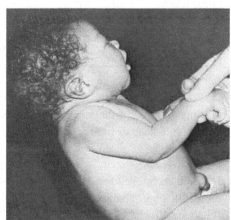

Fig. 3.28. Head lag. Good control. Note ear in line with shoulder and body. Score 4.

Fig. 3.29. Head lag. Excellent head control. Note ear position ahead of shoulder line. Score 5.

VENTRAL SUSPENSION

Method

The infant is suspended in a prone position by a hand under the chest, and the posture of the head, trunk, and limbs is noted (Fig. 3.30).

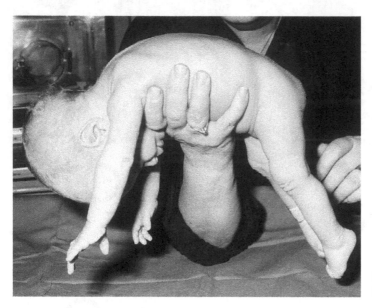

Fig. 3.30. Ventral suspension test.

Scoring ventral suspension test

1	2	3	4	5
back curved, head & limbs hang straight	back curved, head ↓, limbs slightly flexed	back slightly curved, limbs flexed	back straight, head in line, limbs flexed	back straight, head above body

One of the five diagrams is ringed (Fig. 3.31–3.35). If there is discrepancy in head, limb, or trunk posture, the diagram most resembling the trunk posture should be circled, and the deviation of head or limb posture should be drawn on the diagram (Fig. 3.36).

Cautionary tales

Distinctly better head posture in ventral suspension than in the supine position should raise the suspicion of abnormal extensor tone. This item is another one for which the infant's state may affect the response. A sleeping infant, particularly a less mature one, will show a less mature response (a score of 1 or 2, perhaps), whereas a vigorously crying infant, even a very young preterm one, may well have a score of 4.

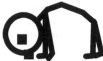

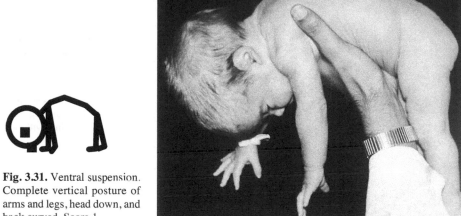

Fig. 3.31. Ventral suspension. Complete vertical posture of arms and legs, head down, and back curved. Score 1.

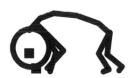

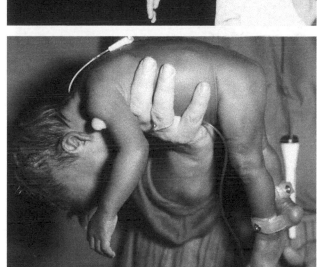

Fig. 3.32. Still pretty floppy, but slight flexion in arms and legs. Score 2.

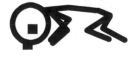

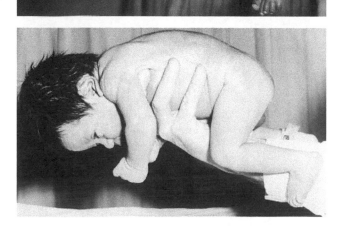

Fig. 3.33. More flexion in arms and legs, back straighter, head almost in line with body. Score 3.

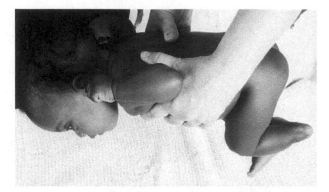

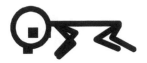

Fig. 3.34. Ventral suspension. Full flexion in arms and legs, back straight, head in line with body. Score 4.

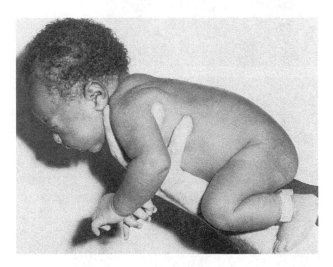

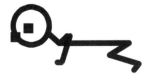

Fig. 3.35. Ventral suspension. Head well above line of body; back straight. Score 5.

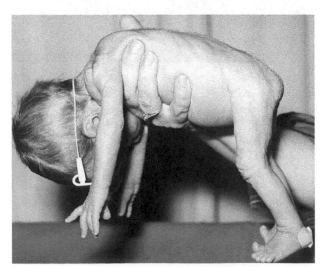

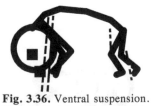

Fig. 3.36. Ventral suspension. Note that back is relatively straight but limbs are straight. If posture does not correspond to any diagram, the one most like posture of back is circled, and deviations of head and/or limbs can be marked.

Tone patterns

Changes in tone in the newborn infant are often generalized. Generalized hypotonia or hypertonia may be a manifestation of a central nervous system (CNS) insult but may also have a systemic cause. In contrast, abnormal tone pattern due to an abnormal distribution of tone is nearly always associated with CNS insult. The abnormal tone patterns commonly observed in the neonate are increased flexor tone in the upper limbs with extensor tone in the lower limbs, a tight popliteal angle relative to the rest of the flexor tone in the legs, and hypertonia of the neck extensors.

Limb tone flexion patterns can be evaluated by comparing leg traction with arm traction, or leg traction with popliteal angle, or simply observing the posture of the arms and legs in the supine infant.

Neck and trunk tone patterns can be evaluated by comparing head flexion with head extension or comparing the amount of extension in head lag and in ventral suspension.

FLEXOR TONE (1) (ON TRACTION: ARMS VERSUS LEGS)
Method
Record the difference between the already circled scores for arm traction and leg traction on page 1 of the proforma. Examples of such comparisons are shown in Fig 3.37.

Scoring flexor tone (1)

1	2	3	4	5
	score for arm flexion less than leg flexion	score for arm flexion equal to leg flexion	score for arm flexion more than leg flexion but difference 1 column or less	score for arm flexion more than leg flexion but difference more than 1 column

Two of the four grades reflect patterns most commonly seen in normal preterm and term infants (columns 2 and 3), while grades 4 and 5 are given for relatively increased flexor tone in the arms.

Cautionary tales
Whereas grade 4 is seen in a small percentage of normal infants and therefore might merely raise some suspicion, grade 5 is always abnormal. Abnormal patterns of leg tone are often observed in infants born in the breech presentation. In such cases, the presentation should be indicated. Abnormal patterns are a consistent feature in infants with bronchopulmonary dysplasia who show shoulder retraction, and are also observed in hyperexcitable infants.

41

	1	2	3	4	5
score on arm traction test is less than on leg traction test (score 2)		arms flex slightly or some resistance felt 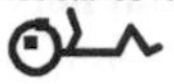 R　　　　L			
			legs flex well till bottom lifts up 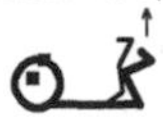 R　　　　L		

	1	2	3	4	5
score on arm traction test is equal to score on leg traction test (score 3)			arms flex well till shoulder lifts, then straighten 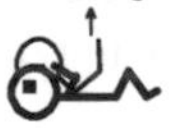 R　　　　L		
			legs flex well till bottom lifts up 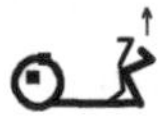 R　　　　L		

	1	2	3	4	5
score on arm traction test is more than on leg traction test, by 1 column only (score 4)			arms flex well till shoulder lifts, then straighten 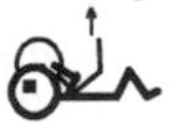 R　　　　L		
		legs flex slightly or some resistance felt 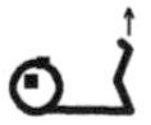 R　　　　L			

	1	2	3	4	5
score on arm traction test is more than on leg traction test, by more than1 column (score 5)				arms flex at approx 100° & maintained as shoulder lifts R　　　　L	
		legs flex slightly or some resistance felt 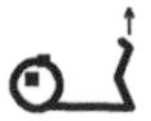 R　　　　L			

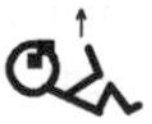

Fig. 3.37. Tone pattern: flexor tone (1). Examples of how to evaluate the difference between arm and leg flexion by comparing the columns circled for arm and leg traction.

FLEXOR TONE (2) (IN SUPINE INFANT: ARMS VERSUS LEGS)
Method
Compare the posture of arms with that of legs in the supine infant.

Scoring flexor tone (2)

1	2	3	4	5
		arms and legs flexed	strong arm flexion with strong leg extension *intermittent*	strong arm flexion with strong leg extension *continuous*

The three grades reflect patterns of distribution seen in preterm and term infants, either normal (grades 3 and 4) or abnormal (grade 5).

Cautionary tales
Abnormal patterns of leg tone are often observed in infants delivered in the breech presentation. In such infants, their presentation at birth should be indicated. Marked increase in arm flexor tone in association with increased leg extensor tone can be observed in normal crying infants. In a quiet infant, regardless of the length of her/his gestation, this pattern should raise the suspicion of CNS pathology. It is, however, non-specific and can be associated with a number of conditions, such as the onset of an intraventricular haemorrhage, hypoxic–ischaemic encephalopathy, and periventricular leukomalacia.

LEG EXTENSOR TONE
Method
Record the difference between the circled scores for popliteal angle and leg traction on page 1 of the proforma. Examples of such comparisons are shown in Fig.3.38.

Scoring leg extensor tone

1	2	3	4	5
	score for leg traction more than score for popliteal angle	score for leg traction equal to score for popliteal angle	score for leg traction less than score for popliteal angle, by 1 column only	score for leg traction less than score for popliteal angle, by more than 1 column

Two of the four grades reflect the patterns of distribution most commonly seen in normal preterm and term infants (columns 2 and 3), while scores of 4 and 5 are given for two grades of relatively tight popliteal angle. No grade 1.

Cautionary tales
Whereas grade 4 is seen in a small percentage of normal infants and therefore might merely raise some suspicion, grade 5 is always abnormal. Abnormal patterns of leg tone are often observed in infants born in the breech presentation, which should therefore be indicated on the chart. A disproportionately tighter popliteal angle than the rest of the leg tone is frequently found in association with germinal matrix or intraventricular haemorrhages.

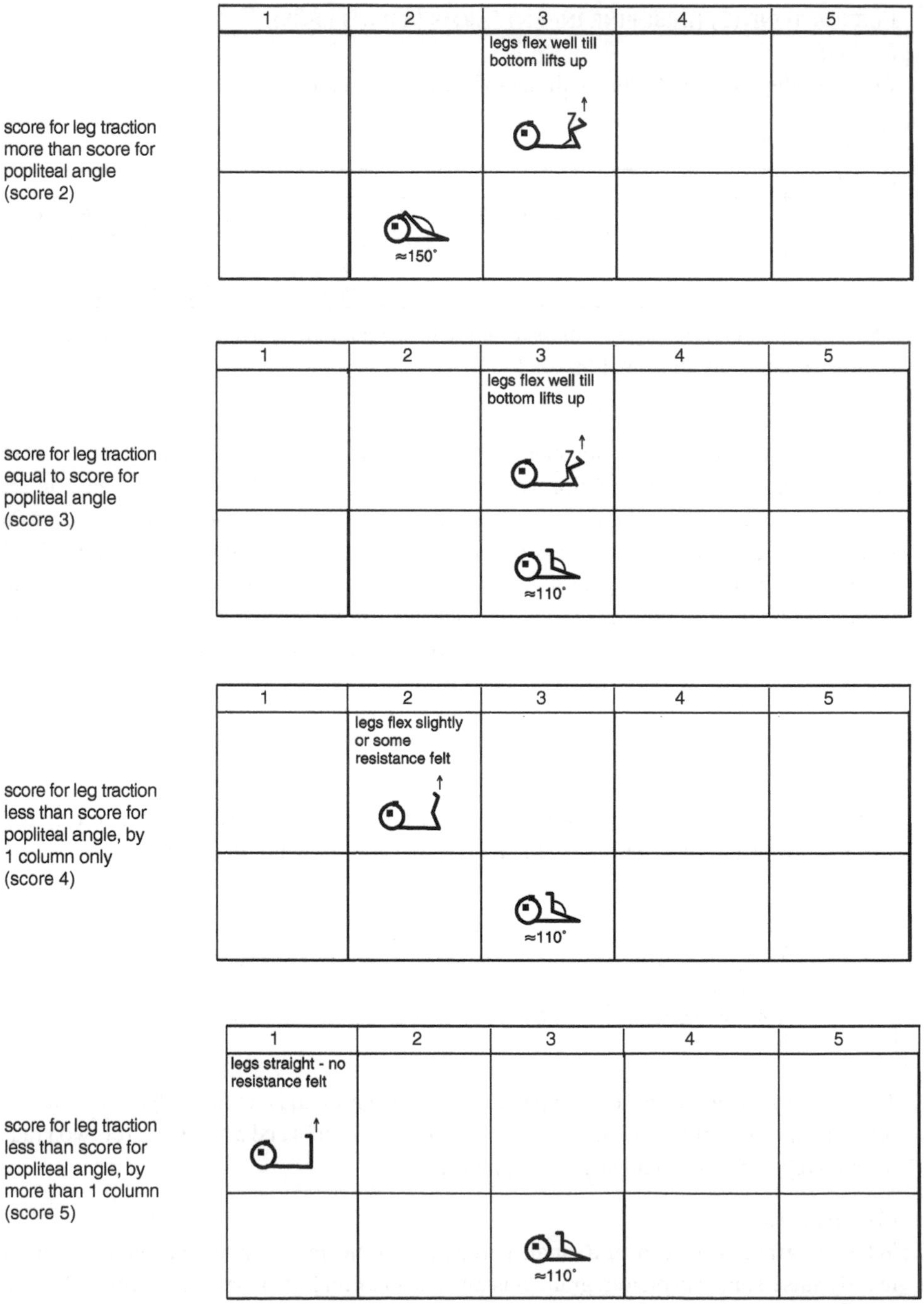

1	2	3	4	5
		legs flex well till bottom lifts up		
	≈150°			

score for leg traction more than score for popliteal angle (score 2)

1	2	3	4	5
		legs flex well till bottom lifts up		
		≈110°		

score for leg traction equal to score for popliteal angle (score 3)

1	2	3	4	5
	legs flex slightly or some resistance felt			
		≈110°		

score for leg traction less than score for popliteal angle, by 1 column only (score 4)

1	2	3	4	5
legs straight - no resistance felt				
		≈110°		

score for leg traction less than score for popliteal angle, by more than 1 column (score 5)

Fig. 3.38. Examples of how to evaluate leg extensor tone by comparing the columns circled for the leg traction test and popliteal angle.

44

NECK EXTENSOR TONE (SITTING)

Method

Record the difference between the already circled scores for head control (1) and head control (2) on page 1 of the proforma. Examples of such comparisons are shown in Fig. 3.39.

Scoring neck extensor tone

1	2	3	4	5
	score for head extension less than head flexion	score for head extension equal to head flexion	score for head extension more than head flexion. but difference 1 column or less	score for head extension more than head flexion but difference more than 1 column

Two of the four grades reflect patterns of distribution most commonly seen in normal preterm and term infants (columns 2 and 3), while scores of 4 and 5 are given for two grades of relatively increased head extension. No grade 1.

Cautionary tales

Whereas grade 4 is seen in a small percentage of normal infants and therefore might merely raise some suspicion, grade 5 is always abnormal. Increased tone of the neck extensormuscles is often associated with hypoxic–ischaemic lesions, meningitis, or increased intraventricular pressure.

ASSESSMENT OF EXTENSOR TONE (HORIZONTAL)

Method

Record the difference between the already circled scores for head lag and ventral suspension on page 1 of the proforma. Examples of such comparisons are shown in Fig. 3.40.

Scoring extensor tone (horizontal)

1	2	3	4	5
	score for ventral suspension less than head lag	score for ventral suspension equal to head lag	score for ventral suspension more than head lag but difference 1 column or less	score for ventral suspension more than head lag but difference more than 1 column

Two of the four grades reflect patterns of distribution most commonly seen in normal preterm and term infants (columns 2 and 3), while scores of 4 and 5 are given for two grades of abnormalities.

Cautionary tales

Whereas grade 4 is seen in a small percentage of normal infants and therefore might merely raise some suspicion, grade 5 is always abnormal. Greater tone of the neck extensor muscles than of the flexor ones is often associated with hypoxic–ischaemic lesions, meningitis, or increased intraventricular pressure.

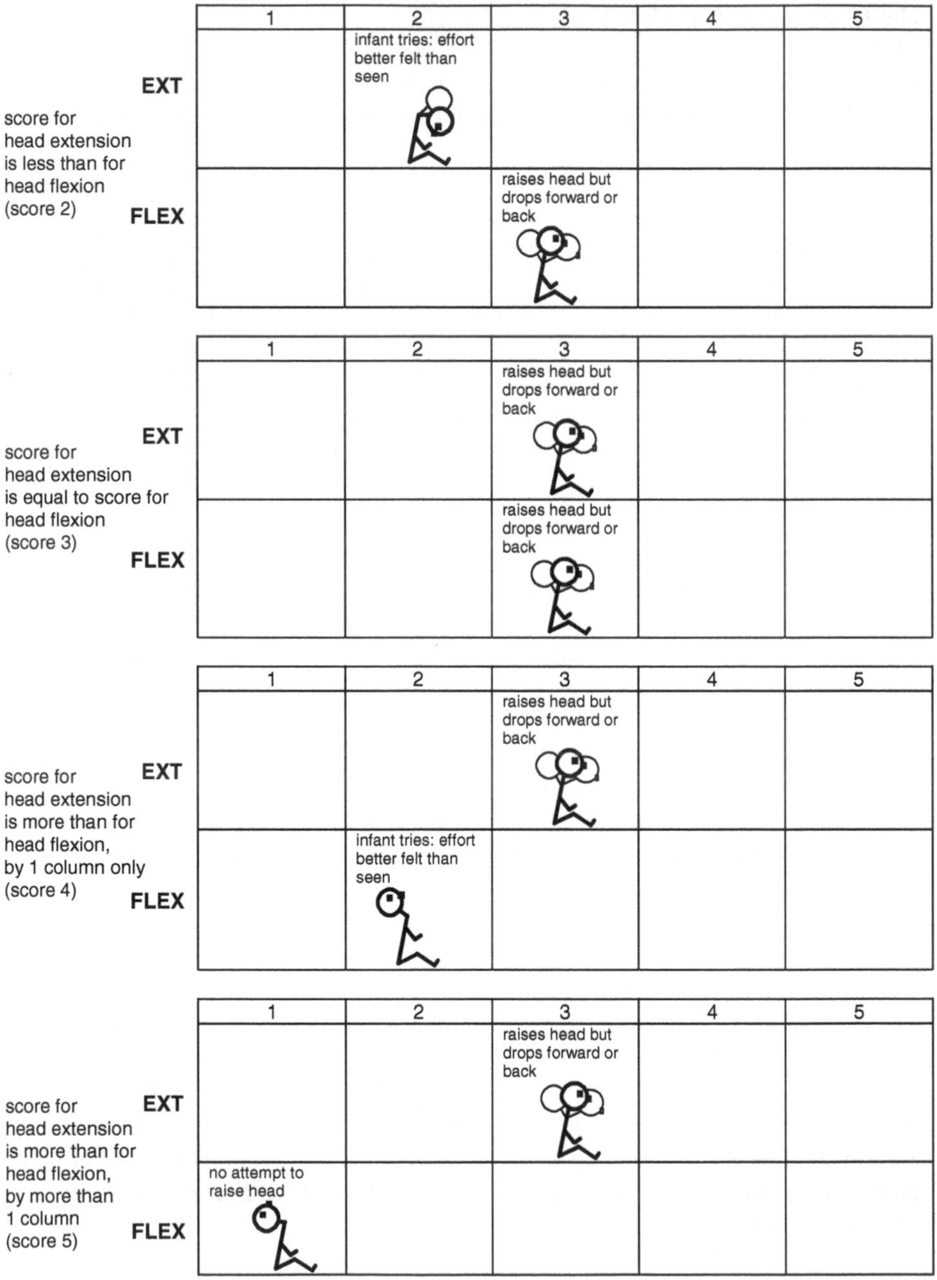

	1	2	3	4	5
EXT		infant tries: effort better felt than seen			
FLEX			raises head but drops forward or back		

score for
head extension
is less than for
head flexion
(score 2)

	1	2	3	4	5
EXT			raises head but drops forward or back		
FLEX			raises head but drops forward or back		

score for
head extension
is equal to score for
head flexion
(score 3)

	1	2	3	4	5
EXT			raises head but drops forward or back		
FLEX		infant tries: effort better felt than seen			

score for
head extension
is more than for
head flexion,
by 1 column only
(score 4)

	1	2	3	4	5
EXT			raises head but drops forward or back		
FLEX	no attempt to raise head				

score for
head extension
is more than for
head flexion,
by more than
1 column
(score 5)

Fig. 3.39. Examples of how to evaluate neck extensor tone by comparing the columns circled for head control (1) (extension) and head control (2) (flexion).

46

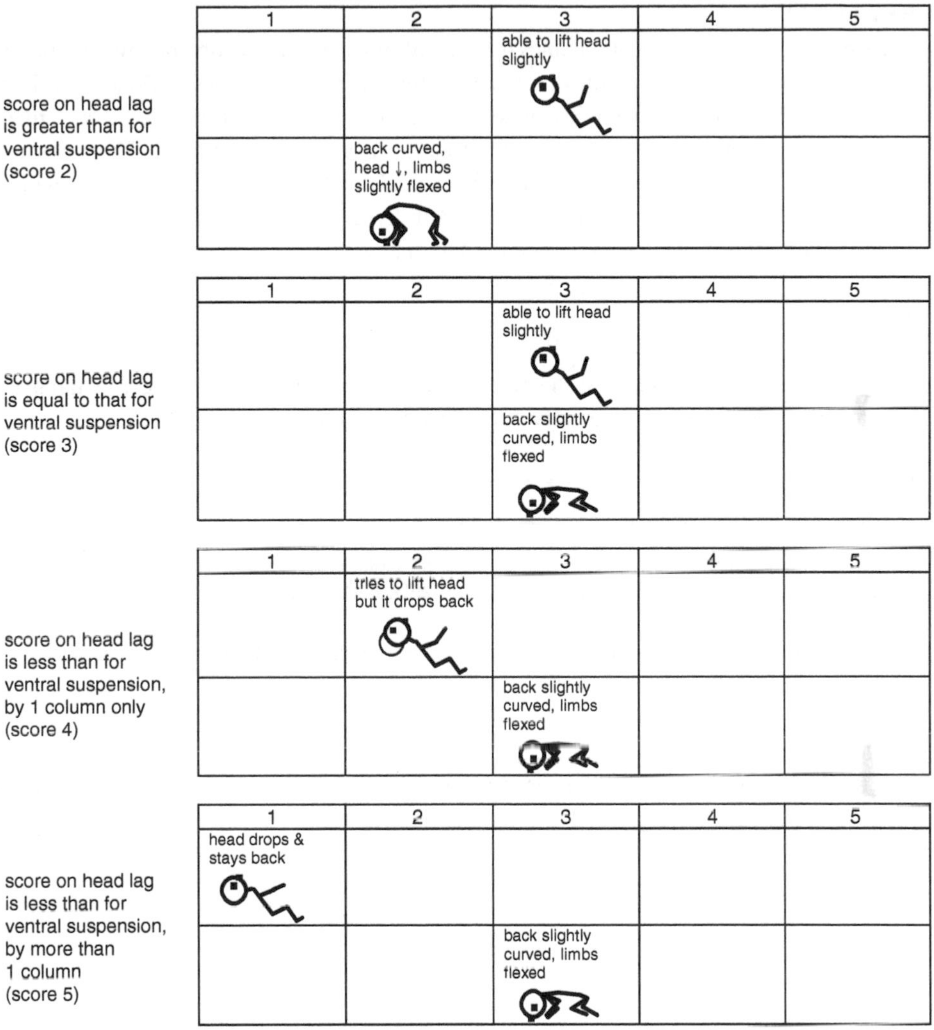

	1	2	3	4	5
score on head lag is greater than for ventral suspension (score 2)			able to lift head slightly		
		back curved, head ↓, limbs slightly flexed			

	1	2	3	4	5
score on head lag is equal to that for ventral suspension (score 3)			able to lift head slightly		
			back slightly curved, limbs flexed		

	1	2	3	4	5
score on head lag is less than for ventral suspension, by 1 column only (score 4)		tries to lift head but it drops back			
			back slightly curved, limbs flexed		

	1	2	3	4	5
score on head lag is less than for ventral suspension, by more than 1 column (score 5)	head drops & stays back				
			back slightly curved, limbs flexed		

Fig. 3.40. Examples of how to evaluate extensor tone (horizontal) by comparing the columns circled for head lag and ventral suspension.

REFLEXES

It has been traditional for most schemes for the neurological examination of newborn infants to include large numbers of primitive reflexes. Although interesting, these reflexes contribute little to the detection of neurological abnormalities in the newborn infant, and indeed many of them are present in anencephalic and other grossly abnormal infants. Their possible value lies in their asymmetry in certain pathological conditions, their absence in generally unresponsive infants, and their low threshold in hyperresponsive infants. From the vast inventory of reflexes, we have retained the few that we think are the most useful.

TENDON REFLEXES

Method

With the infant lying supine, test the biceps, knee, and ankle jerks with a gentle tap using a small patella hammer or, especially in preterm infants, just the finger.

Scoring tendon reflexes

1	2	3	4	5
absent	felt, not seen	seen	"exaggerated" (very brisk)	clonus

The five categories are: absent; felt, not seen; seen; exaggerated; and clonus (scored from 1 to 5, respectively).

Cautionary tales

Any of these grades could occur in isolation in a perfectly normal infant; conversely, a grossly abnormal infant can have perfectly normal tendon reflexes.

SUCK/GAG REFLEX

Method

This reflex is assessed by placing an index finger (pad towards palate) in the mouth of the infant, and documenting the rhythmicity and strength of the sucking response (Fig. 3.41).

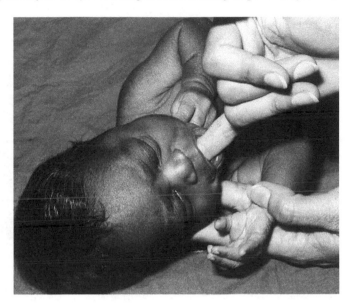

Fig. 3.41. Testing suck/gag reflex.

Scoring the suck/gag reflex

1	2	3	4	5
no gag / no suck	weak irregular suck only	weak regular suck	strong suck: (a) irregular (b) regular	no suck but strong clenching
	No stripping	Some stripping	Good stripping	

We have defined four sequential grades and have added a fifth (scored 5) which is aberrant and characterized by a firm clenching but no regular sucking movement.

Cautionary tales

We are unsure whether grade 5 is an exaggerated or a diminished response. Some infants may clench initially, and suck rhythmically only subsequently, when stimulated by movement of the finger: for these we have ringed two separate grades. Although weak or abnormal sucking is often a sign of neurological abnormality, regular, strong sucking may also occur in the presence of gross neurological abnormality (contrary to the common belief, particularly among nursing staff, that normal sucking is a sign of infant well-being). We have added to the proforma the absence of a gag reflex, which we would test only if the sucking response is absent.

PALMAR GRASP

Method

The infant should be lying supine with the head in midline. Each side is tested, separately or together, by placing an index finger in the palm of the hand (Fig. 3.42).

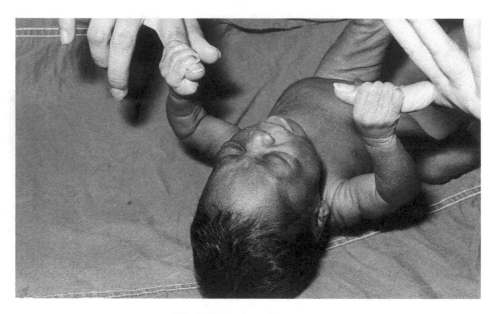

Fig. 3.42. Testing palmar grasp.

Scoring palmar grasp

1	2	3	4	5
no response	short, weak flexion of fingers	strong flexion of fingers	strong finger flexion, shoulder ↑	very strong grasp; infant can be lifted off couch
R L	R L	R L	R L	R L

The five grades are shown in order of increasing response. Score any asymmetries.

Cautionary tales

Do not touch the dorsum of the infant's hand, as this may inhibit the grasp response. The optimal state for the response is 3, 4, or 5, and by this stage of the examination the infant is usually in one of those states.

PLANTAR GRASP

Method

The infant should be supine with the head in the midline. The two sides are stimulated simultaneously by placing a thumb under the ball of each foot, underneath the toes. The response is the curling of the toes over the examiner's fingers (Fig. 3.43, left).

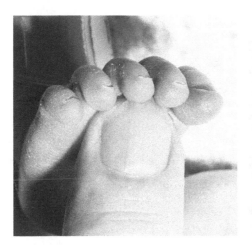 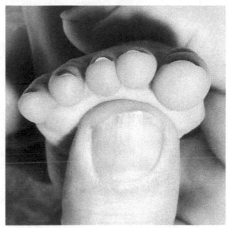

Fig. 3.43. Testing plantar grasp. (Left) Infant's toes curve around examiner's finger. (Right) No plantar flexion of infant's toes around examiner's fingers.

Scoring plantar grasp

1	2	3	4	5
no response	short, weak flexion of fingers	strong flexion of fingers	strong finger flexion, shoulder ↑	very strong grasp; infant can be lifted off couch
R　　　　L	R　　　　　L	R　　　　　L	R　　　　　L	R　　　　　L

The three grades of increasing response are shown. Score any asymmetries.

Cautionary tales

Do not touch the dorsum of the foot, as this will produce dorsiflexion of the toes. Asymmetry of this response is often found in association with brain lesions contralateral to the weaker response.

PLACING REFLEX

Method

The infant is held upright by encircling her/his chest under the arms with both hands. Stroke the front of the infant's leg with the edge of the table or other examining surface (Fig. 3.44).

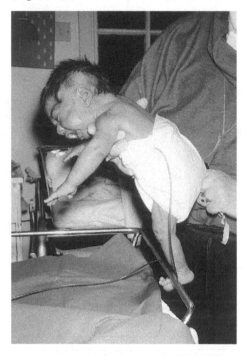

Fig. 3.44. Testing the placing reflex.

Scoring the placing reflex

1	2	3	4	5
no response	dorsiflexion of ankle only	full placing response with flexion of hip and knee & placing sole on surface		
R L	R L	R L		

The response is scored according to the degree of flexion of the leg.

MORO REFLEX

Method

When the infant's condition permits, we prefer to elicit the Moro reflex by the "head drop" method. The infant is held suspended in a supine position raised at 45° with one hand behind the upper back and the other supporting the head; her/his arms should be over the chest. The head is held in a midline position and dropped back about 10° (Fig. 3.45). The response is graded on the basis of the arm movements only, and the test may be repeated two or three times to get a detailed observation.

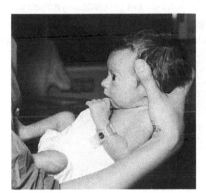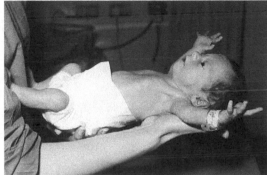

Fig. 3.45. Testing the Moro reflex.

Scoring the Moro reflex

1	2	3	4	5
no response, or opening of hands only	full abduction at shoulder and extension of the arms; no adduction	full abduction, but only delayed or partial adduction	partial abduction at shoulder, and extension of arms followed by smooth adduction	• minimal abduction or adduction • no abduction or adduction; only forward extension of arms • marked adduction only

Grade 1 is complete lack of response, or opening of the hands only. Grade 2 is full abduction at the shoulders and extension of the arms at the elbows, but no adduction at the shoulders or flexion of the elbows. Grade 3 is full abduction at the shoulders and extension of the arms, but only partial or delayed adduction with minimal arm flexion at the elbows. Grade 4 is partial abduction and extension, followed by good adduction and flexion of the arms.

53

Grade 5 is seen in some infants who show only marked adduction of the arms across the chest, and in others in whom there is practically no abduction or there is adduction at the shoulders, with the predominant response being extension of the arms only at the elbows and elevation of the arms. Grade 5 also provides for scoring a Moro reponse with a high threshold (difficult to elicit) and producing only a minimal adduction and/or abduction.

Cautionary tales

Grade 5 includes some responses that can be normal variants but are more commonly associated with CNS insults. Asymmetry of the Moro reflexes will be produced by lower motor neuron lesions, whereas upper motor neuron lesions do not produce asymmetry. In infants with impaired consciousness or with basal ganglia lesions, it can be quite difficult to elicit this reflex. Therefore, the threshold at which the reflex can be elicited should also be noted.

NORMAL AND ABNORMAL MOVEMENTS

SPONTANEOUS MOVEMENTS

Method

Observe the supine infant. Note spontaneous movements for a couple of minutes, preferably while the infant is awake and quiet. Both the quality and quantity of spontaneous movements are observed in order to evaluate the patterns and the sequence of movements of the whole body, rather than concentrating on single segments, such as arms or legs.

Scoring spontaneous movements

The quantity and the quality of movements are scored separately.

1	2	3	4	5
no movement	sporadic and short isolated movements	frequent isolated movements	frequent generalized movements	continuous exaggerated movements

Quantity. 5 grades are described, ranging from the absence of movements to the presence of exaggerated movements.

1	2	3	4	5
	hands open, toes straight most of the time	intermittent fisting or thumb adduction	continuous fisting or thumb adduction; index finger flexion, thumb opposition	continuous big toe extension or flexion of all toes

Quality. These responses could be placed in various sequences, but we have tried to reflect the sequence of maturation of normal movements in the first three columns, leaving columns 4 and 5 for two degrees of abnormal movements. Grade 1 includes the predominant presence of stretches, mainly found in very preterm infants (below 32 weeks). Grade 2 includes more mature patterns where jerky movements and stretches still persist but fluent alternating movements are also observed. The latter progressively become the prevalent pattern as the infant approaches term age (column 3). Fluent movements can be described as smooth movements involving all parts of the body, head, trunk, legs, and arms in a continuous way without interruptions and showing good variability and complexity, with subtle fluctuations of amplitude and speed. The observer notes not only the movements of flexion and extension of the limbs, but also more subtle movements, such as changes in direction of the movements and slight rotations that make them more "elegant". Grades 4 and 5 include some abnormal patterns of movements such as monotonous ones, in which the sequence varies little, or other abnormal patterns where the movements are not fluent but are repetitive or brisk and chaotic. It also includes *cramped, synchronized* movements in which all limb and trunk muscles contract and relax at the same time, and other abnormal movements such as mouthing.

Cautionary tales

Movements should be observed at the beginning of the examination and ideally should be scored when the infant is quiet. If there is no opportunity to see the infant in the ideal state, the observation should be scored and the infant's state clearly noted.

HEAD RAISING IN PRONE POSITION

Method

The infant is placed prone with the head in the midline, and the movements of the head are noted over a period of about 30 seconds.

Scoring head raising in prone position

1	2	3	4	5
no response	infant rolls head over, chin not raised	infant raises chin, rolls head over	infant brings head and chin up	infant brings head up and keeps it up

One of the five grades of response is circled.

Cautionary tales

This item is very state dependent; however, prolonged head raising by an infant in a quiet state should raise a suspicion of increased extensor tone.

ABNORMAL SIGNS/PATTERNS

Under this heading is included a series of abnormal signs that are not related to maturation, graded roughly in relation to their persistence and severity.

ABNORMAL HAND OR TOE POSTURES

Method

The infant is observed in the supine position. The predominant posture of fingers and toes is noted.

Scoring abnormal hand or toe postures

1	2	3	4	5
	hands open, toes straight most of the time	intermittent fisting or thumb adduction	continuous fisting or thumb adduction; index finger flexion, thumb opposition	continuous big toe extension or flexion of all toes

The four grades compare the most normal position (column 2) and a normal variant (column 3) with abnormal positions of fingers (column 4) and toes (column 5). The abnormal positions that should be noted in particular are: abnormal thumb and fisting (Fig. 3.46) and other unusual hand postures such as opposition of the thumb and index finger with the other three fingers extended (Fig. 3.47). The abnormal foot postures include spontaneously up-going toes (spontaneous Babinski) (Fig. 3.48) and the posture of the feet when all toes curl under (flexion of toes) (Fig. 3.49).

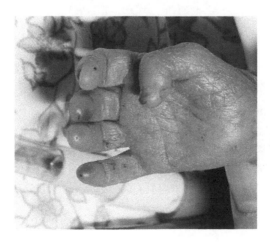

Fig. 3.46. Abnormal hand posture showing thumb adduction.

57

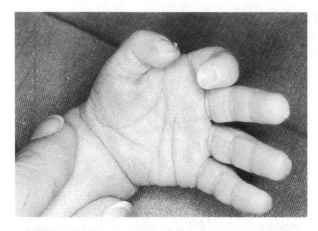

Fig. 3.47. Abnormal hand posture showing opposition of index finger and thumb, with the other three fingers extended.

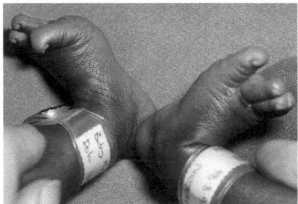

Fig. 3.48. Spontaneously upgoing toes.

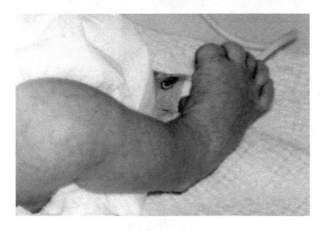

Fig. 3.49. All toes curling under.

Cautionary tales
Some of the abnormal finger and toe positions may occur in a vigorously crying infant.

TREMOR
Method
The infant is observed throughout the whole examination. The presence of tremors or other abnormal movements is noted.

Scoring tremor

1	2	3	4	5
	no tremor, or tremor only when crying or only after Moro reflex	tremor occasionally when awake	frequent tremors when awake	continuous tremors

The scoring strip shows four grades.

Cautionary tales
In the earlier edition of this manual we tried to record the incidence, frequency, and amplitude of tremors during the examination, in a method similar to Prechtl's. In practice, we have found that a number of less experienced observers had difficulties in defining a slow or fast response and recorded these randomly. The recording of amplitude has been excluded in this version.

STARTLE
Method
The infant is observed throughout the whole examination. The presence of startles or other abnormal movements is noted.

Scoring startle

1	2	3	4	5
no startle even to sudden noise	no spontaneous startle but reacts to sudden noise	2-3 spontaneous startles	more than 3 spontaneous startles	continuous startles

The incidence of startles over the course of the examination is recorded as one of five grades.

ORIENTATION AND BEHAVIOUR
Neurobehavioural items

From the Brazelton neurobehavioural assessment scheme we selected some items that we thought most likely to reflect the infants's neurological status, rather than inherent temperament. In order to conform with the rest of our neurological scheme, we deviated from Brazelton's scoring system and adapted these items to our 5-point scale, grading the responses according to increasing intensity. We have also added two items – eye movements and quality of the infant's cry – that are not strictly neurobehavioural but that we commonly observe while doing the neurobehavioural examination.

EYE APPEARANCES

Method

The spontaneous eye movements of the awake infant are observed. The character and symmetry of eye movements are also noted in response to stimulation with a red ball or target.

Scoring eye appearances

1	2	3	4	5
does not open eyes		full conjugated eye movements	*transient* • nystagmus • strabismus • roving eye • movements • sunset sign	*persistent* • nystagmus • strabismus • roving eye • movements abnormal pupils

The sequence of the four categories is not particularly significant, except that columns 4 and 5 probably represent two grades of the most significantly abnormal sign.

Cautionary tales

The "sunset sign" (see column 4), usually thought to be a sign of raised intracranial tension, commonly occurs in normal preterm infants approaching 40 weeks postmenstrual age, especially if dolicocephalic, and the sign is often absent in infants with rapidly progressive ventricular enlargement. Nystagmus may be seen in normal newborn infants but is relatively rare as a manifestation of neurological disease in this age group.

AUDITORY ORIENTATION

Method

We use a rattle with a broad band (white noise) of approximately 60 to 80 dB rather than the human voice, as it is more practical when testing infants inside incubators. The infant is elevated about 20° in the supine and the head is supported in the midline by the examiner's hand, leaving it free to rotate. The auditory stimulus is presented on each side in turn, with the examiner's hand and the rattle out of sight, at a distance of about 10 cm inside an incubator or about 15 to 25 cm outside (Fig. 3.50).

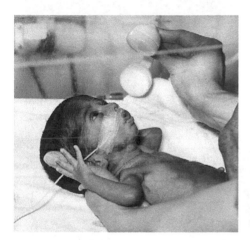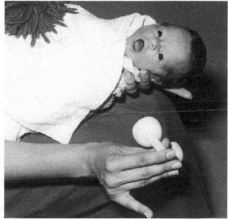

Fig. 3.50. Testing auditory orientation.

Scoring auditory orientation

1	2	3	4	5
no reaction	auditory startle; brightens and stills; no true orientation	shifting of eyes, head might turn towards source	prolonged head turn to stimulus; search with eyes; smooth	turns head and eyes towards noise every time but jerky abrupt

The five grades of response reflect the infant's ability to respond to and localize the source of the stimulus. Note any asymmetry (Fig. 3.51).

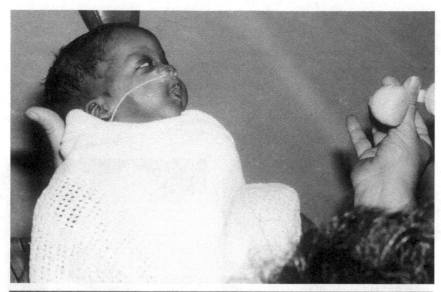

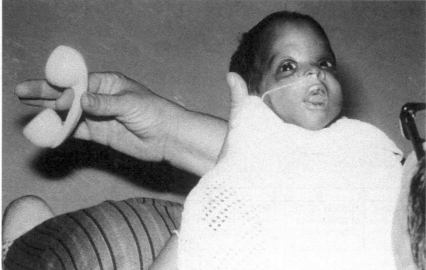

Fig. 3.51. Hearing response to rattle. The infant has a good response (eye and head turning) to the left (a) but not to the right (b). Testing for auditory brain stem response at this time showed normal response to 60 dB on the left but doubtful response on the right.

Cautionary tales

A strong visual stimulus may inhibit the auditory response of a visually alert infant, and, on the other hand, a visual cue from a rattle can produce an apparently positive response in a deaf infant. A good response is probably significant even under difficult environmental conditions, but a poor response in an incubator or other noisy environment should be interpreted with caution.

VISUAL ORIENTATION

Method

We have found that a red woollen ball is an excellent stimulus for infants of all gestational ages and is easy to handle inside or outside an incubator (Fig. 3.52). A black-and-white target is also a good stimulus. The infant is tested in a propped-up supine position (as for auditory orientation) and the stimulus is presented at a distance of 15 to 25cm, starting in the midline and moving laterally in either direction, then vertically, and finally in an arc. The infant's ability to focus and fixate on the object and to track (follow) it is assessed.

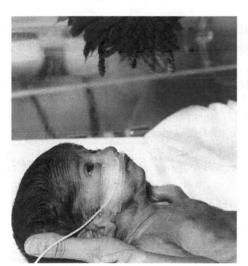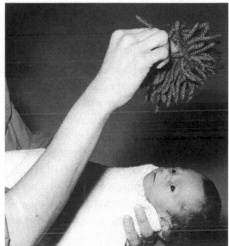

Fig. 3.52. Testing visual orientation.

Scoring visual orientation

1	2	3	4	5
does not follow or focus on stimuli	stills, focuses, follows briefly to the side but loses stimuli	follows horizontally and vertically; no head turn	follows horizontally and vertically; turns head	follows in a circle
B T	B T	B T	B T	B T

The response is graded from 1 to 5.

Cautionary tales

Several difficulties have been encountered that may interfere with successful assessment and its interpretation.

• The human face may distract the infant, and the mother watching from the side within the infant's view, or the examiner's face, may inhibit the response to the test object. This is particularly likely to occur in the more alert infant, and we have observed it frequently in the preterm infant reaching 40 weeks postmenstrual age. (This may explain the inability of some observers to document the good tracking one can obtain with these infants.)

- Hyperactive infants, especially if small for dates, may inhibit their visual activity when exhibiting a lot of random arm movements. This may be overcome by swaddling the infant to restrain the arm movements.

- Bright ambient lighting, especially fluorescent lighting, which is so common in neonatal nurseries, may inhibit the visual responses of infants, who frequently do not open their eyes fully in such circumstances. These infants are much more responsive when the lights are switched off and they are assessed in a state of semi-darkness. This again stresses the importance of environmental factors in many of the responses of newborn infants.

- While normal infants show a good reaction to both the red ball and the target, there are some in whom one of the two stimuli can be less effective. The cause is still unclear but we recommend using both stimuli.

- Unfortunately, in contrast to previous claims (Miranda and Hack 1979), visual function that is apparently good cannot be regarded as a proof of an intact visual pathway or as a marker of future neurological integrity. Infants with peripheral retina lesions due to retrolental fibroplasia can track. However, these lesions may later affect more central parts of the retina and cause blindness. Also, infants with extensive subcortical cystic leukomalacia apparently affecting the occipital lobe may also have excellent tracking abilities in the neonatal period, which disappear at around 48 to 52 weeks postmenstrual age, confirming that early vision is not necessarily cortically mediated (Dubowitz et al. 1986). On the other hand, infants with an intact occipital cortex but basal ganglia lesions are unable to fixate and follow the target (Mercuri et al. 1997).

ALERTNESS
Method
This is tested as response to visual stimuli (red ball or target).

Scoring alertness

1	2	3	4	5
will not respond to stimuli	when awake, looks only briefly	when awake, looks at stimuli but loses them	keeps interest in stimuli	does not tire (hyper-reactive)

We have based our grading on the quality of responses to the visual stimuli or the ease with which the orientation responses are elicited.

Cautionary tales
Alertness should be based not on the infant's appearance but on the ability to respond to stimulation. Staring eyes, for instance, may give the appearance of hyperalertness in moderately asphyxiated infants and in apnoeic infants treated with theophylline, although these infants may respond poorly to stimuli.

IRRITABILITY

This has been adapted from Brazelton's "peak of excitement". This item measures the infant's overall responsiveness to the examination: her/his ability to become aroused and to reach a state of intense motor activity and crying, and then to revert to a lower state, either spontaneously or by the examiner consoling her/him. Basically, it is also a reflection of the variability of the infant's state in the course of the examination.

Scoring irritability

1	2	3	4	5
quiet all the time, not irritable to any stimuli	awakes, cries sometimes when handled	cries often when handled	cries always when handled	cries even when not handled

We have subdivided the response into five grades.

Cautionary tales

Irritability is scored as a response to being handled. Therefore, only the irritability occurring during the examination should be recorded. If the infant was irritable on other occasions but not during the examination, this should be noted separately but not scored.

CONSOLABILITY

This measures the infant's ability to be consoled once she/he has reached a crying state, either spontaneously or by various manoeuvres carried out by the examiner.

1	2	3	4	5
not crying; consoling not needed	cries briefly; consoling not needed	cries; becomes quiet when talked to	cries; needs picking up to be consoled	cries; cannot be consoled

Irritability and consolability, considered together, will give a clear reflection of the infant who is unresponsive, apathetic, and difficult to rouse, or the infant who is overresponsive, hyperirritable, and difficult to console. Either pattern can reflect an abnormal neurological state.

CRY

This item has been included to document the quantity and quality of the infant's cry during the examination. It may prove a useful index of abnormality when the cry is diminished or excessive or altered in character.

Scoring cry

1	2	3	4	5
no cry at all	whimpering cry only	cries to stimuli but normal pitch		High-pitched cry; often continuous

Four possible scores are given.

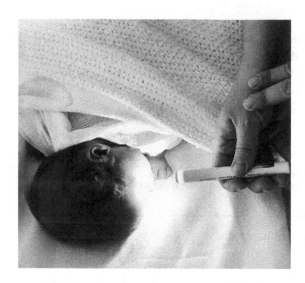

Fig. 3.53. Testing habituation to light.

Additional items (optional) – Habituation

Habituation reflects the decrease in a response to repetitive stimuli.

HABITUATION TO LIGHT

This is the first test done, and the child is left undisturbed and preferably asleep. We use a standard optometric torch (Fig. 3.53), which gives a bright, well-defined circle of light. Successive stimuli are applied, with an intervening gap of about 5 seconds, and two consecutive negative responses are taken as a shutdown. In most infants the response (either blinking or body movement) is brief, and 5 seconds is adequate for the infant to quieten again before the next stimulus is applied. In some infants whose response is prolonged, it may be necessary to wait longer than 5 seconds. If the reaction continues longer than 20 seconds, we abandon the test, as the length between stimuli then becomes too long for them to be considered repetitive.

Instead of Brazelton's nine grades of response, we classify the responses in five broad grades, as follows:

(1) No response, even in state 2.

(2) Variable or unclassifiable responses, including (a) a blink response to the first stimulus only, and then no further response; (b) a tonic blink response, that is, a sustained closure of the eyes in response to a single stimulus and lasting as long as 30 seconds or even more, and with very slow relaxation (as discussed above, further stimulation is then no longer feasible); (c) variable response to the repetitive stimuli, with vacillation in type of response and difficulty in fitting it into any consistent category. (Subdivisions a, b, and c are arbitrary; they are merely grouped together for convenience and are not incremental.)

(3) Response to repetitive stimuli (blink and/or body movement) and shutdown within five stimuli (i.e. no response for two consecutive stimuli after the fifth stimulus, or earlier).

(4) Response to repetitive stimuli and shutdown within 10 stimuli.

(5) Response to repetitive stimuli but no shutdown by the 10th stimulus. We also include in this grade infants who have come to a fully awake state by the 10th stimulus, which we look upon as increased responsiveness (or low threshold) to stimulation.

Habituation to light can be assessed in infants from 27 or 28 weeks gestation, but in general, infants under 31 weeks often exhibit the tonic type of response.

HABITUATION TO SOUND

For this test we use the "telephone" rattle supplied with the Denver test kit, or a similar commercial one (see Fig. 3.50). It has a wide frequency band and can be stopped quickly. However, we have recently observed that glass beads in a universal container bottle are equally effective. For this test we uncover the infant so that leg movements can be observed, but do not wake her/him. Our basic grading (which, again, is adapted from the original Brazelton method) is along similar lines to the habituation to light:

(1) No response even in state 2.

(2) (a) Slight movement in response to first stimulus only and no further response.

(b) Variable response to successive stimuli and difficult to fit into any consistent category.

(3) Startle or movement in response to two to five stimuli, followed by complete shutdown.

(4) Startle or movement in response to 6 to 10 stimuli, followed by shutdown.

(5) We have grouped together in this category the infant who responds to 10 successive stimuli, with no shutdown on the 11th; the infant who comes to a fully awake state in the course of the first 10 stimuli; and the infant who shows startles or major responses throughout the test.

Particular note should be taken if there is no response at all on more than one separate occasion, particularly if the infant is in state 2, as this may reflect hearing loss. We consider a poor response on habituation more significant than a poor response to auditory orientation.

The habituation to sound tends to show marked day-to-day variation in the same infant, except possibly at the two extremes of response, and it may be extremely difficult to test, because the infant may not be in a suitable state when examined or may change state during the examination. Nevertheless, we have found this item to be a useful one to include in the routine neurological assessment. It helps to identify the unresponsive deaf infant and the hyperresponsive irritable infant, and is also a useful means of gradually waking the sleeping infant and getting her/him into a suitable state for the rest of the assessment.

After completion of the habituation testing, the infant is gently undressed. If she/he is attached to infusions or monitoring equipment it is unnecessary to remove all the clothing; usually it is adequate merely to uncover the infant and loosen various garments as appropriate and feasible.

4
THE NEUROLOGICAL PROFILE OF NORMAL PRETERM AND TERM INFANTS

In this chapter we discuss the neurological signs observed in the normal preterm infant at various gestational ages and the postnatal maturation of these signs, and we compare some of them at 40 weeks postmenstrual age with those in the newborn normal term infant. It is beyond the scope of this manual to give details of all the cumulative data on each item in the assessment scheme, and we have thus selected some items that, in our experience, best illustrate the type of information obtainable using this approach. The scheme has provided a baseline for detecting deviations in some of the signs in preterm infants with known neurological abnormality, enabling us to diagnose specific abnormalities on the basis of these deviations. Later (in Chapter 6) we describe how to apply the method to the evaluation of preterm infants with brain lesions, such as intraventricular haemorrhage or periventricular leukomalacia, and show how deviations in clinical signs, both initially and during postnatal maturation, may relate to pathological events in the central nervous system.

Maturation of the preterm infant
The maturation of neurological items was assessed longitudinally in a population of 57 preterm infants whose gestational ages at birth were 28 to 35 weeks. The infants were assessed within 7 days of birth and again at 40 weeks postmenstrual age. The findings on this second examination are compared with those for 35 term infants examined on days 1 and 5.

Posture and tone
Most of the neurological items assessing posture and tone are age dependent, reflecting the increase in flexor tone in the limbs and the increase in axial tone with increasing maturity. Figures 4.1 to 4.4 illustrate some examples of tone and posture recorded in normal infants at 28, 32, 36, and 40 weeks.

Figs. 4.1–4.4 *(pages 69–72)*. Examples of evolution of posture and tone with gestational age. These were recorded in preterm infants (gestational ages 28, 32, or 36–37 weeks; Figs. 4.1–4.3, respectively) and term infants (gestational age 40 weeks; Fig. 4.4). Note that these are only examples and there may be some variability.

28 weeks

POSTURE Infant supine. Look mainly at position of legs but also note arms. *Score predominant posture.*	arms & legs extended or very slightly flexed	legs slightly flexed	legs well flexed but not adducted	legs well flexed & adducted near abdomen	abnormal posture: a) opisthotonus b) marked leg extension, strong arm flexion
ARM RECOIL Take both hands, quickly extend arms parallel to the body, Count to three. Release. Repeat 3 times.	arms do not flex	arms flex slowly, not always; not completely	arms flex slowly; more completely	arms flex quickly and completely	arms difficult to extend; snap back forcefully
ARM TRACTION Hold wrist and pull arm upwards. Note flexion at elbow and resistance while shoulder lifts off table. *Test each side separately.*	arms remain straight; no resistance felt	arms flex slightly or some resistance felt	arms flex well till shoulder lifts, then straighten	arms flex at approx 100° & maintained as shoulder lifts	flexion of arms <100°; maintained when body lifts up
LEG RECOIL Take *both* ankles in one hand, flex hips + knees. Quickly extend. Release. Repeat 3 times.	No flexion	incomplete or variable flexion	complete but slow flexion	complete fast flexion	legs difficult to extend; snap back forcefully
LEG TRACTION Grasp ankle and slowly pull leg upwards. Note flexion at knees and resistance as buttocks lift. *Test each side separately.*	legs straight - no resistance felt	legs flex slightly or some resistance felt	legs flex well till bottom lifts up	knee flexes remains flexed when bottom up	flexion stays when back+bottom up
POPLITEAL ANGLE Fix knee on abdomen, extend leg by gentle pressure with index finger behind the ankle. Note angle at knee. *Test each side separately.*	180°	≈150°	≈110°	~90°	<90°
HEAD CONTROL (1) *(extensor tone)* Infant sitting upright. Encircle chest with both hands holding shoulders. Let head drop forward.	no attempt to raise head	infant tries: effort better felt than seen	raises head but drops forward or back	raises head: remains vertical; it may wobble	
HEAD CONTROL (2) *(flexor tone)* Infant sitting upright. Encircle chest with both hands holding shoulders. Let head drop backward.	no attempt to raise head	infant tries: effort better felt than seen	raises head but drops forward or back	raises head: remains vertical; it may wobble	head upright or extended; cannot be passively flexed
HEAD LAG Pull infant towards sitting posture by traction on both wrists & support head slightly. Also note arm flexion.	head drops & stays back	tries to lift head but it drops back	able to lift head slightly	lifts head in line with body	head in front of body
VENTRAL SUSPENSION Hold infant in ventral suspension. Observe back, flexion of limbs, and relation of head to trunk. If it looks different, DRAW.	back curved, head & limbs hang straight	back curved, head ↓, limbs slightly flexed	back slightly curved, limbs flexed	back straight, head in line, limbs flexed	back straight, head above body

32 weeks

POSTURE Infant supine. Look mainly at position of legs but also note arms. *Score predominant posture.*	arms & legs extended or very slightly flexed	legs slightly flexed	legs well flexed but not adducted	legs well flexed & adducted near abdomen	abnormal posture: a) opisthotonus b) marked leg extension, strong arm flexion
ARM RECOIL Take both hands, quickly extend arms parallel to the body, Count to three. Release. Repeat 3 times.	arms do not flex	arms flex slowly, not always; not completely	arms flex slowly; more completely	arms flex quickly and completely	arms difficult to extend; snap back forcefully
ARM TRACTION Hold wrist and pull arm upwards. Note flexion at elbow and resistance while shoulder lifts off table. *Test each side separately.*	arms remain straight; no resistance felt	arms flex slightly or some resistance felt	arms flex well till shoulder lifts, then straighten	arms flex at approx 100° & maintained as shoulder lifts	flexion of arms <100°; maintained when body lifts up
LEG RECOIL Take *both* ankles in one hand, flex hips + knees. Quickly extend. Release. Repeat 3 times.	No flexion	incomplete or variable flexion	complete but slow flexion	complete fast flexion	legs difficult to extend; snap back forcefully
LEG TRACTION Grasp ankle and slowly pull leg upwards. Note flexion at knees and resistance as buttocks lift. *Test each side separately.*	legs straight - no resistance felt	legs flex slightly or some resistance felt	legs flex well till bottom lifts up	knee flexes remains flexed when bottom up	flexion stays when back+bottom up
POPLITEAL ANGLE Fix knee on abdomen, extend leg by gentle pressure with index finger behind the ankle. Note angle at knee. *Test each side separately.*	180°	≈150°	≈110°	≈90°	<90°
HEAD CONTROL (1) *(extensor tone)* Infant sitting upright. Encircle chest with both hands holding shoulders. Let head drop forward.	no attempt to raise head	infant tries: effort better felt than seen	raises head but drops forward or back	raises head: remains vertical; it may wobble	
HEAD CONTROL (2) *(flexor tone)* Infant sitting upright. Encircle chest with both hands holding shoulders. Let head drop backward.	no attempt to raise head	infant tries: effort better felt than seen	raises head but drops forward or back	raises head: remains vertical; it may wobble	head upright or extended; cannot be passively flexed
HEAD LAG Pull infant towards sitting posture by traction on both wrists & support head slightly. Also note arm flexion.	head drops & stays back	tries to lift head but it drops back	able to lift head slightly	lifts head in line with body	head in front of body
VENTRAL SUSPENSION Hold infant in ventral suspension. Observe back, flexion of limbs, and relation of head to trunk. If it looks different, DRAW.	back curved, head & limbs hang straight	back curved, head ↓, limbs slightly flexed	back slightly curved, limbs flexed	back straight, head in line, limbs flexed	back straight, head above body

Fig. 4.2. *(Caption on page 68)*

36-37 weeks

POSTURE Infant supine. Look mainly at position of legs but also note arms. *Score predominant posture.*	arms & legs extended or very slightly flexed	legs slightly flexed	legs well flexed but not adducted	legs well flexed & adducted near abdomen	abnormal posture: a) opisthotonus b) marked leg extension, strong arm flexion
ARM RECOIL Take both hands, quickly extend arms parallel to the body, Count to three. Release. Repeat 3 times.	arms do not flex	arms flex slowly; not always; not completely	arms flex slowly; more completely	arms flex quickly and completely	arms difficult to extend; snap back forcefully
ARM TRACTION Hold wrist and pull arm upwards. Note flexion at elbow and resistance while shoulder lifts off table. *Test each side separately.*	arms remain straight; no resistance felt	arms flex slightly or some resistance felt	arms flex well till shoulder lifts, then straighten	arms flex at approx 100° & maintained as shoulder lifts	flexion of arms <100°; maintained when body lifts up
LEG RECOIL Take *both* ankles in one hand, flex hips + knees. Quickly extend. Release. Repeat 3 times.	No flexion	incomplete or variable flexion	complete but slow flexion	complete fast flexion	legs difficult to extend; snap back forcefully
LEG TRACTION Grasp ankle and slowly pull leg upwards. Note flexion at knees and resistance as buttocks lift. *Test each side separately.*	legs straight - no resistance felt	legs flex slightly or some resistance felt	legs flex well till bottom lifts up	knee flexes remains flexed when bottom up	flexion stays when back+bottom up
POPLITEAL ANGLE Fix knee on abdomen, extend leg by gentle pressure with index finger behind the ankle. Note angle at knee. *Test each side separately.*	180°	≈ 150°	≈110°	≈90°	<90°
HEAD CONTROL (1) *(extensor tone)* Infant sitting upright. Encircle chest with both hands holding shoulders. Let head drop forward.	no attempt to raise head	infant tries: effort better felt than seen	raises head but drops forward or back	raises head: remains vertical; it may wobble	
HEAD CONTROL (2) *(flexor tone)* Infant sitting upright. Encircle chest with both hands holding shoulders. Let head drop backward.	no attempt to raise head	infant tries: effort better felt than seen	raises head but drops forward or back	raises head: remains vertical; it may wobble	head upright or extended; cannot be passively flexed
HEAD LAG Pull infant towards sitting posture by traction on both wrists & support head slightly. Also note arm flexion.	head drops & stays back	tries to lift head but it drops back	able to lift head slightly	lifts head in line with body	head in front of body
VENTRAL SUSPENSION Hold infant in ventral suspension. Observe back, flexion of limbs, and relation of head to trunk. If it looks different, DRAW.	back curved, head & limbs hang straight	back curved, head ↓, limbs slightly flexed	back slightly curved, limbs flexed	back straight, head in line, limbs flexed	back straight, head above body

Fig. 4.3. *(Caption on page 68)*

71

40 weeks

POSTURE Infant supine. Look mainly at position of legs but also note arms. *Score predominant posture.*	arms & legs extended or very slightly flexed	legs slightly flexed	legs well flexed but not adducted	legs well flexed & adducted near abdomen	abnormal posture: a) opisthotonus b) marked leg extension, strong arm flexion
ARM RECOIL Take both hands, quickly extend arms parallel to the body, Count to three. Release. Repeat 3 times.	arms do not flex	arms flex slowly, not always; not completely	arms flex slowly; more completely	arms flex quickly and completely	arms difficult to extend; snap back forcefully
ARM TRACTION Hold wrist and pull arm upwards. Note flexion at elbow and resistance while shoulder lifts off table. *Test each side separately.* R L	arms remain straight; no resistance felt	arms flex slightly or some resistance felt	arms flex well till shoulder lifts, then straighten	arms flex at approx 100° & maintained as shoulder lifts	flexion of arms <100°; maintained when body lifts up
LEG RECOIL Take *both* ankles in one hand, flex hips + knees. Quickly extend. Release. Repeat 3 times.	No flexion	incomplete or variable flexion	complete but slow flexion	complete fast flexion	legs difficult to extend; snap back forcefully
LEG TRACTION Grasp ankle and slowly pull leg upwards. Note flexion at knees and resistance as buttocks lift. *Test each side separately.* R L	legs straight - no resistance felt	legs flex slightly or some resistance felt	legs flex well till bottom lifts up	knee flexes remains flexed when bottom up	flexion stays when back+bottom up
POPLITEAL ANGLE Fix knee on abdomen, extend leg by gentle pressure with index finger behind the ankle. Note angle at knee. *Test each side separately.* R L	180°	≈150°	≈110°	≈90°	<90°
HEAD CONTROL (1) *(extensor tone)* Infant sitting upright. Encircle chest with both hands holding shoulders. Let head drop forward.	no attempt to raise head	infant tries: effort better felt than seen	raises head but drops forward or back	raises head: remains vertical; it may wobble	
HEAD CONTROL (2) *(flexor tone)* Infant sitting upright. Encircle chest with both hands holding shoulders. Let head drop backward.	no attempt to raise head	infant tries: effort better felt than seen	raises head but drops forward or back	raises head: remains vertical; it may wobble	head upright or extended; cannot be passively flexed
HEAD LAG Pull infant towards sitting posture by traction on both wrists & support head slightly. Also note arm flexion.	head drops & stays back	tries to lift head but it drops back	able to lift head slightly	lifts head in line with body	head in front of body
VENTRAL SUSPENSION Hold infant in ventral suspension. Observe back, flexion of limbs, and relation of head to trunk. If it looks different, DRAW.	back curved, head & limbs hang straight	back curved, head ↓, limbs slightly flexed	back slightly curved, limbs flexed	back straight, head in line, limbs flexed	back straight, head above body

Fig. 4.4. *(Caption on page 68)*

72

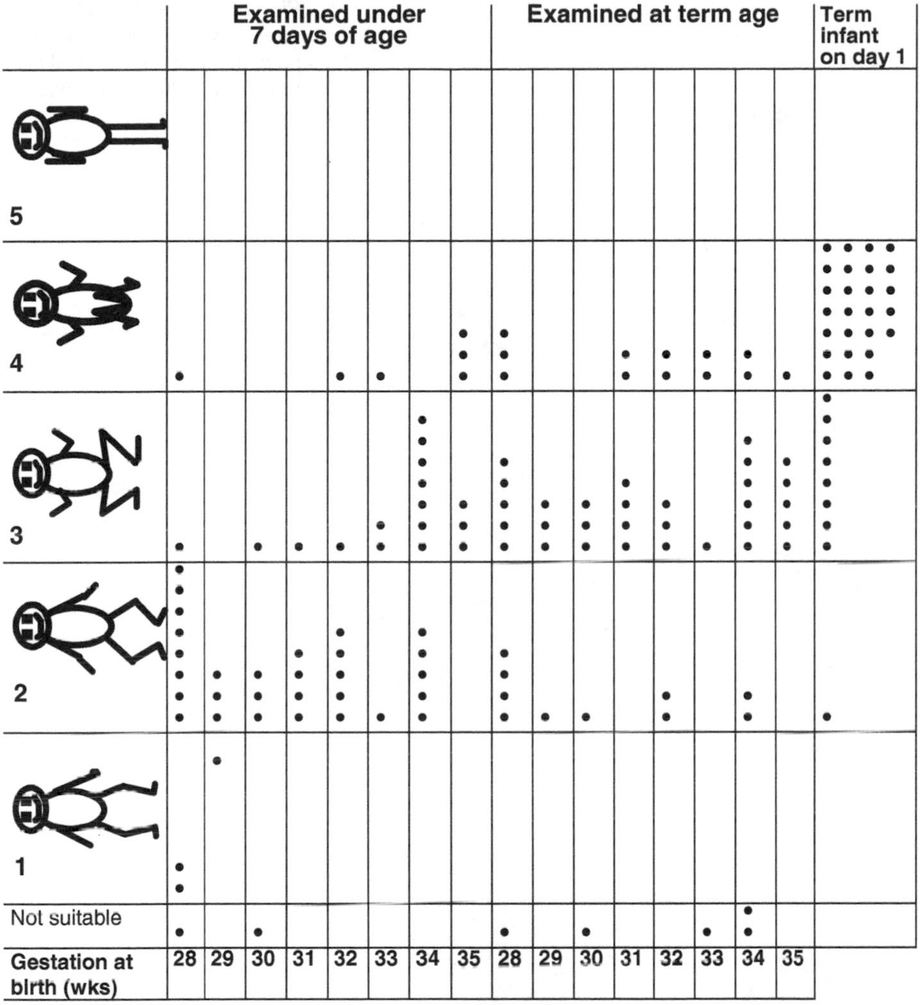

	Examined under 7 days of age								Examined at term age								Term infant on day 1

Gestation at birth (wks): 28 29 30 31 32 33 34 35 | 28 29 30 31 32 33 34 35

Posture categories (top to bottom): 5, 4, 3, 2, 1, Not suitable.

Fig. 4.5. Observed evolution of posture in 57 preterm infants of various gestational ages examined in first postnatal week and at term age. Findings for term newborn infants examined on day 1 are shown in right-hand column for comparison.

● represents one infant.

POSTURE

With increasing maturity, the infant passes from a predominantly extended posture, through one with extension in the upper limbs but flexion in the lower limbs, to one with flexion in both upper and lower limbs, and eventually to one with flexion and adduction in all four limbs. The range of gestational or postmenstrual ages at which each posture occurs is fairly wide. Although these preferential postures are also often difficult to define, particularly at lower postmenstrual ages, when the infant tends to exhibit a lot of random movements, they are nevertheless distinct and consistent enough to be easily recordable in a drowsy infant. The maturation of posture is summarized in Figure 4.5. Most of the preterm infants born

73

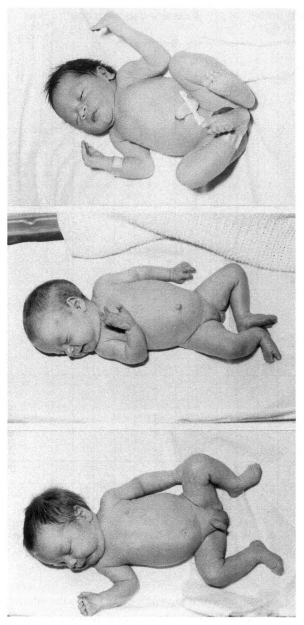

Fig. 4.6. Comparison of posture in term newborn infant (top) and preterm infants (gestational ages 28 [middle] and 29 [bottom] weeks), on reaching term age.

at less than 32 weeks gestational age initially showed a predominantly extended posture (grade 1) and those born at 33 to 35 weeks showed a partially flexed posture. Twenty-six of the 35 term infants showed a fully flexed posture of the arms and legs (grade 4) on day 1. Only a few term infants showed a more extended position.

A distinct difference, however, was noted between the postures of term infants on day 1 and preterm infants on reaching 40 weeks postmenstrual age (Fig. 4.6). Most of the preterm infants, on reaching term age, had only partially flexed posture and often had an asymmetrical tonic neck reflex (posture 2). This posture was most noticeable in infants with the shortest gestation and in the ones who spent most of their time in the prone position, suggesting an effect of extrauterine environment. These infants had a distinctly different posture from that of infants who were mainly cared for in the supine position, who tended to show more abduction of the hips. Interestingly, a posture of very flexed arms, with or without extension of the legs, was not noted in our sample of normal preterm infants at 40 weeks postmenstrual age, suggesting that this posture is abnormal in this population.

LIMB TONE
The traction response and recoil both increase with gestational age, reflecting the increase in flexor tone with increasing maturity. This is well illustrated by the response to arm traction, which showed very poor arm flexion at 28 to 30 weeks (grade 1) and progressively increased with gestational age. A similar progression was seen with regard to leg traction, arm recoil, and leg recoil. At 40 weeks postmenstrual age, the flexor tone in the preterm infants was less marked than in the term infants on day 1, as illustrated in Figure 4.7. Of the 38 term infants, 37 showed a good arm flexion response (grade 3, 4, or 5) and only one showed a grade-1 or grade-2 response, whereas more than half of the preterm infants showed this response and few had the fully mature response. All the preterm infants at 40 weeks postmenstrual age also showed less leg flexion than newborn term infants. The reduction in flexor tone at 40 weeks postmenstrual age was more marked in the arms than in the legs.

Trunk and neck tone
Flexor tone of the neck muscles can be seen in newborn infants from about 28 weeks gestation, but it is not evident in the pull-to-sit manoeuvre until several weeks later. In normal infants, good extensor tone in the neck muscles often cannot be seen until they have reached term age. Low-risk (but not high-risk) preterm infants have better head control at 40 weeks postmenstrual age than newborn term infants (Palmer et al. 1982)

The maturation of the extensor tone can be well illustrated by the infant's posture in ventral suspension.

VENTRAL SUSPENSION
In ventral suspension, as the infant's axial extensor tone increases with increasing maturity, the back becomes less rounded, and the head is held more in line with the body. In contrast, both the upper and lower limbs show increased flexion, due to increasing flexor tone in the limbs. Figure 4.8 illustrates the very curved back, complete head drop, and straight limbs seen on this test in most of the infants born at 32 weeks or less. Of infants born at 32 to 35 weeks, an increasing proportion showed less curvature of the back, better head control, and more flexed limbs. Two-thirds scored grade 2 and one-third scored grade 3. The majority of term infants were able to maintain some degree of extension of the head and back on day 1, with the arms and legs partially flexed (a score of 2 on this test). However, when the preterm infants were reassessed at 40 weeks postmenstrual age, a substantial number had better head and trunk posture (a score of 4) than the term infants, but their limbs, unlike

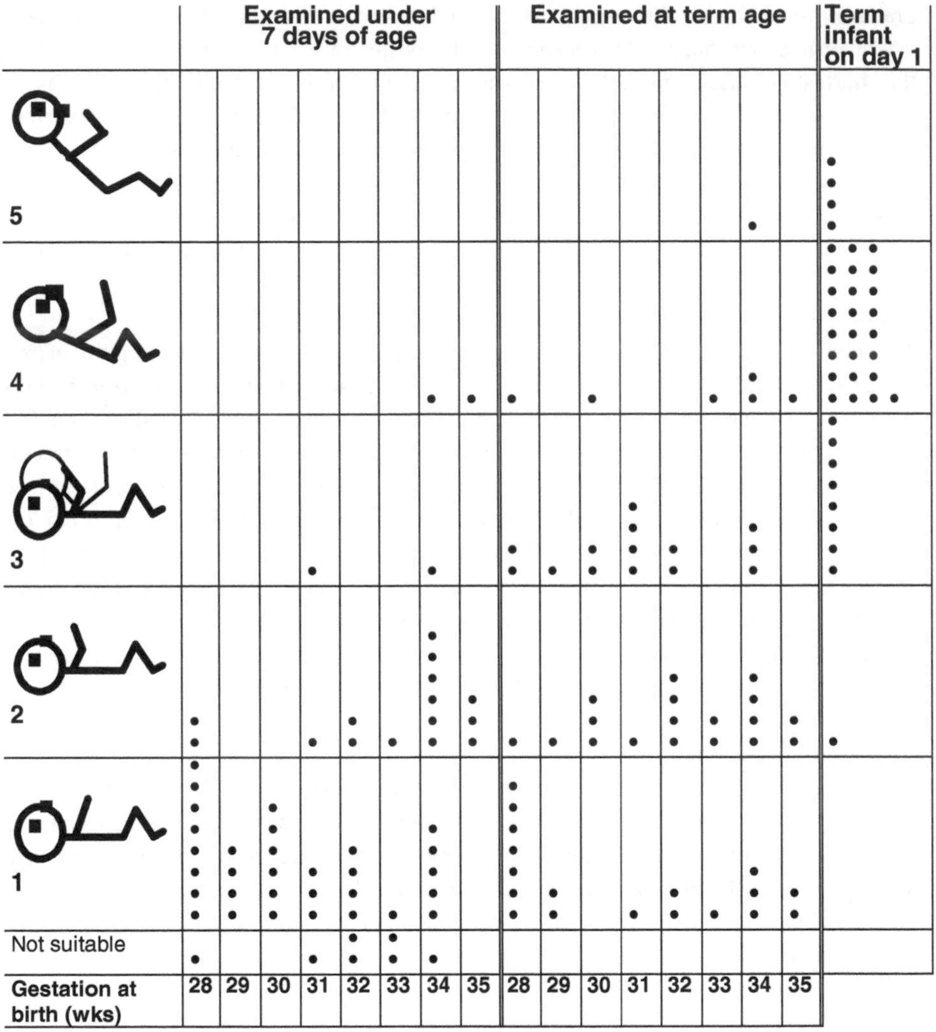

Fig. 4.7. Observed evolution of response to arm traction in preterm infants of various gestational ages at birth, examined in first week of life and at term age. Term newborn infants examined on day 1 are shown in right-hand column for comparison.
● represents one infant.

those of the term infants, were often extended (indicated on the chart by a distinct symbol) (Figs. 4.8 and 4.9). Even in those infants with poorer head or trunk extension (grade 2 or 3), the legs were often extended. It is important to recognize this difference in the posture of the preterm infant at 40 weeks postmenstrual age as being part of the normal pattern of development outside the uterus, in contrast to the flexed posture of the term infant, and not to regard it as a sign of "spasticity".

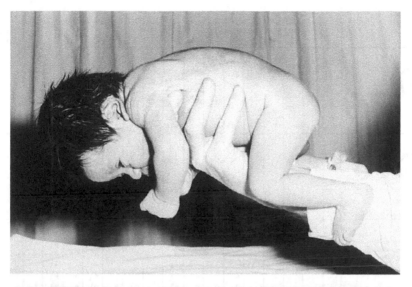

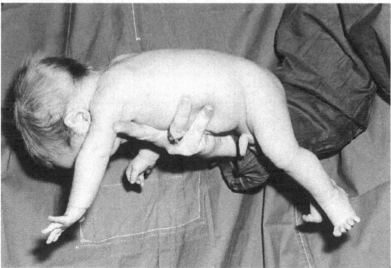

Fig. 4.8. Comparison of response to ventral suspension in a term newborn infant (top) and in a preterm infant born at 28 weeks' gestational age (bottom), on reaching term age.

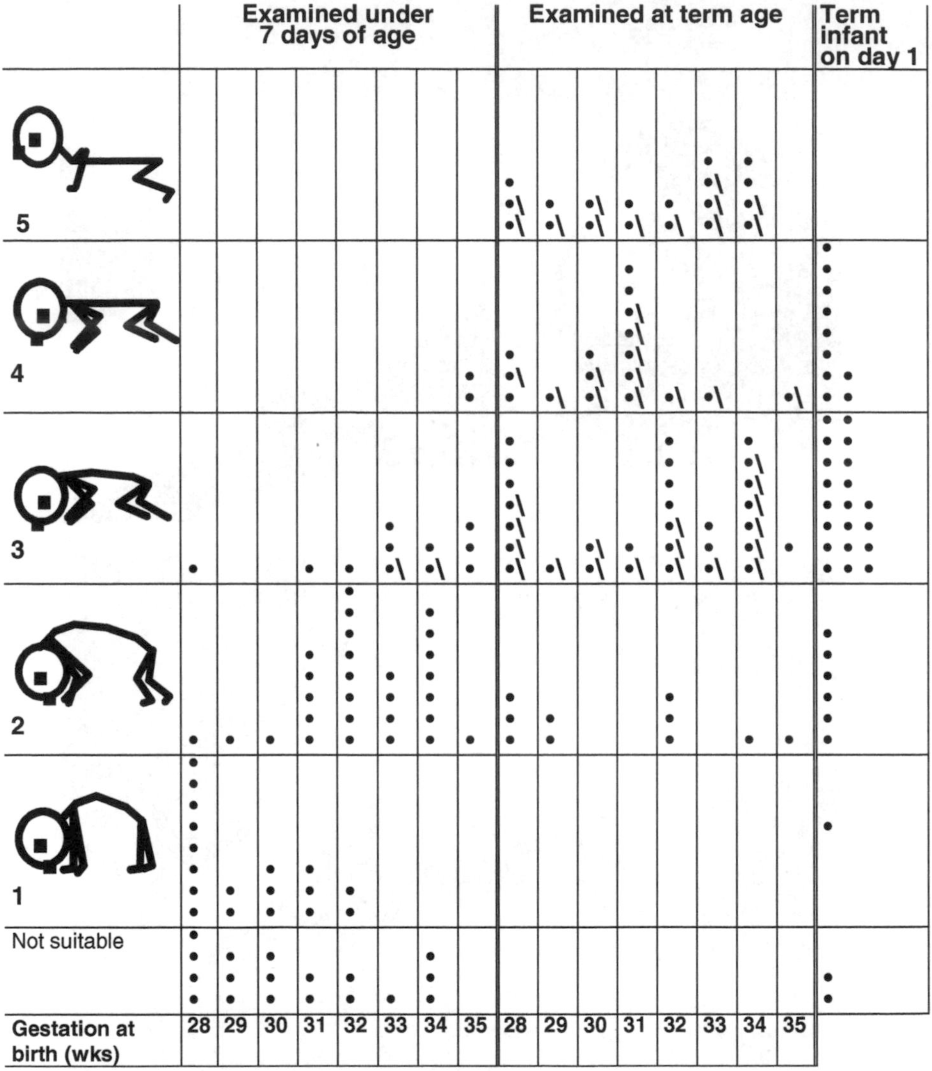

	Examined under 7 days of age	Examined at term age	Term infant on day 1

5

4

3

2

1

Not suitable

| Gestation at birth (wks) | 28 | 29 | 30 | 31 | 32 | 33 | 34 | 35 | 28 | 29 | 30 | 31 | 32 | 33 | 34 | 35 | |

Fig. 4.9. Observed evolution of response to ventral suspension in preterm infants of various gestational ages at birth, examined in first week of life and at term age. Scores for term newborn infants examined on day 1 are shown in right-hand column for comparison.

● represents one infant; ●\, infant also extended legs.

78

Movements

Both the quality and the quantity of spontaneous movements change with increasing gestational age. Movements in preterm infants often consist of slow, asymmetrical twisting and stretching of the trunk and limbs. This may be accompanied by rapid, repetitive wide-amplitude movements of the limbs, resembling myoclonus. There is a gradual change with increasing gestational age to smooth, alternating arm movements with medium speed and intensity. The quantity of motor activities differs little in infants at postmenstrual ages of 28 to 35 weeks and decreases rapidly thereafter, whether the infant is maturing inside or outside the uterus.

Reflexes

A multitude of transitory reflexes that are unique to the neonate have been described. Many of them are already present in early gestation and show a distinctive developmental profile.

PALMAR GRASP

Stimulation of the palm of the hand produces weak flexion of the fingers from 27 or 28 weeks postmenstrual age. With increasing maturity, the contraction spreads to the arm, until at 37 to 38 weeks this is strong enough to allow the infant's shoulder to be lifted off the couch.

PLANTAR GRASP

Plantar grasp is already developed in infants of 26 weeks postmenstrual age and becomes only slightly stronger with increasing maturity.

SUCK/GAG

A sucking reflex is already present at 27 to 28 weeks gestation. With increasing maturity sucking becomes more powerful and better coordinated with swallowing, and by 32 to 34 weeks, a normal infant can feed orally. With the development of sucking and swallowing, there is also a characteristic feeding posture. It has been shown that the maturation of oral feeding is more related to postnatal than to postmenstrual age (Casaer et al. 1982).

PLACING

An attempt to place the foot after a stimulus to its dorsum can already be seen from 34 weeks postmenstrual age and matures to the full response in the next 2 to 4 weeks.

MORO REFLEX

Figure 4.10 illustrates the maturation of the Moro reflex with increasing gestational age. At 25 to 27 weeks gestational age, the only response is the opening of the hand. With increasing maturity, extension and abduction of the upper extremity can be seen, followed by some adduction at the shoulder from 33 to 34 weeks postmenstrual age. The adduction gradually becomes stronger. Abduction and adduction are equal in term infants at birth, and in the next few weeks the adduction becomes weaker. However, the maturation of this response is very different inside the uterus from that outside it. Optimal preterm infants show much less adduction at 40 weeks postmenstrual age than term infants.

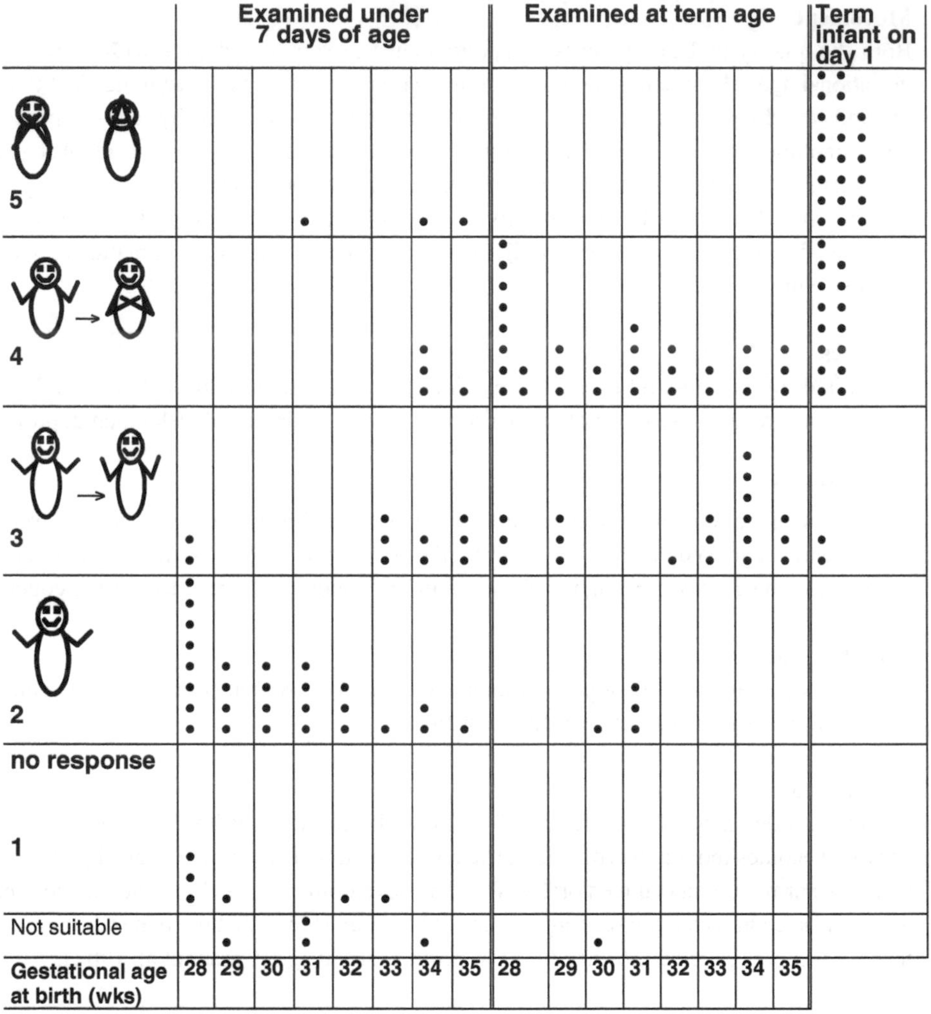

Fig. 4.10. Observed evolution of Moro reflex in preterm infants of various gestational ages at birth, examined in first week of life and at term age. Scores for term newborn infants examined on day 1 are shown in right-hand column for comparison.

● represents one infant.

Behaviour

VISUAL ORIENTATION

In the past, it was thought that the ability to track a visual target develops only after birth. However, in our neurological examination of even very young preterm infants, we have found that even before 32 weeks gestation, some could already focus on a red woollen ball, though they could not yet track its movement. After 32 weeks, many of them could track horizontally or vertically, and some even in an arc. When assessed at 40 weeks postmenstrual age, almost all the preterm infants could visually track the ball, most of them vertically as well as horizontally, and a substantial fraction also in an arc. This performance in the preterm infants reaching term was far better than that in the newborn term infants (Fig. 4.11). These findings are contrary to those published by other authors (Kurtzberg et al. 1979) and may be due to environmental factors. In our unit we encourage low ambient lighting, because we have observed that infants often do not open their eyes in the presence of strong fluorescent lighting but will open them immediately when these are switched off.

AUDITORY ORIENTATION

A response to an auditory stimulus can already be elicited in neurologically normal infants from 27 to 28 weeks postmenstrual age. This response is reliable and correlates well with the presence of an auditory brainstem response (ABR). A poor response, however, particularly in a noisy environment, should be treated with caution, as 20 to 30% of infants with a normal ABR may have an absent clinical response.

Evolution of neurological signs in term infants in the first week of life

When term infants were assessed on day 1 and again at the end of the first week of life, we noted that no or little change was observed for some items, such as ventral suspension, whereas for others, more marked changes were observed (Fig. 4.12). In particular, we noted a decrease in the degree of flexion as shown by a less flexed posture and a decrease of flexor tone in the limbs. We also noted a clear improvement in visual orientation. While on day 1 there was still a fair proportion of term infants who could only focus or at best could briefly follow horizontally, by day 5 most of these infants could track both horizontally and vertically, and a few in an arc as well.

Small size for gestational age

Infants who at birth are small for their gestational age (SGA) often show a neurological profile different from that of term infants whose weight at birth is appropriate for their gestational age. SGA infants have often been described in the past as apathetic and hypotonic (Schulte et al. 1971, Als et al. 1976). These observations, however, were usually made in infants born to mothers with preeclampsia who had received medication in late pregnancy and during delivery. A different picture emerged from the assessment of SGA infants born at term of an uncomplicated pregnancy and labour and whose mothers had received no medication (Dubowitz et al. 1983). Soon after birth, these infants were found to be hypertonic and hyperalert, to have a low threshold for primitive reflexes, and to habituate poorly. Often the sucking response was tonic and the Moro reflex consisted of an extension reaction

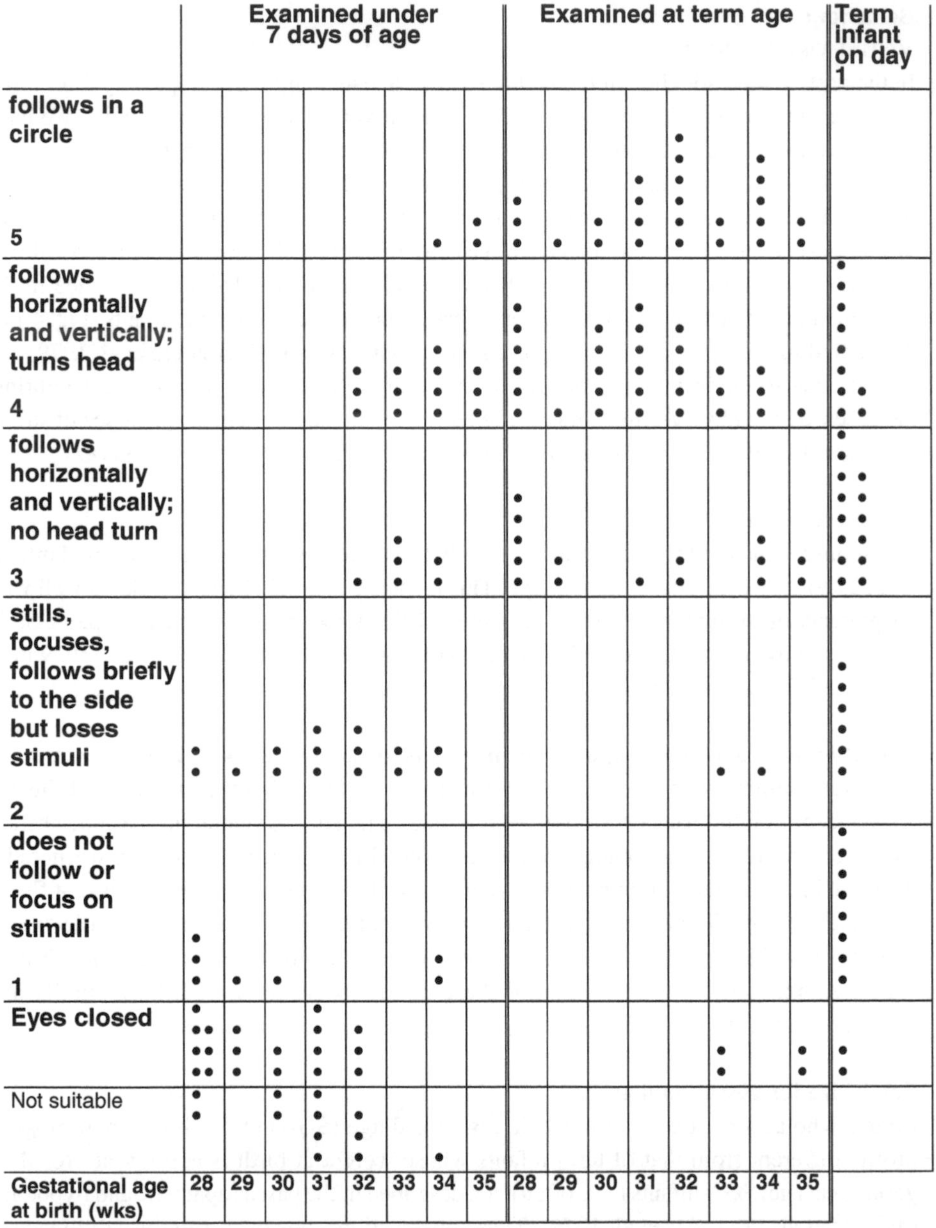

	Examined under 7 days of age								Examined at term age								Term infant on day 1
follows in a circle 5						•	•	••	••• •	•	•	•	•••• 	•	•••• 	•	•
follows horizontally and vertically; turns head 4			•••	••	•••	••	•	•	•••• 	•	••	•••	••	•	•	•	•••• • •
follows horizontally and vertically; no head turn 3					•••	•	•		•••• 	••		•	•		••	•	• •• •• •• •• ••
stills, focuses, follows briefly to the side but loses stimuli 2	••	•	••	•••	•••	•	•							•	•		••••••
does not follow or focus on stimuli 1	•••	•	•		••												•••••••
Eyes closed	•••• ••	•••	••	••• 	••									•		•	•
Not suitable	•• 		•• 	• ••	••• 	•											
Gestational age at birth (wks)	28	29	30	31	32	33	34	35	28	29	30	31	32	33	34	35	

Fig. 4.11. Evolution of visual orientation in preterm infants of various gestational ages examined in first week and at term age. Term newborn infants examined on day 1 are shown in right-hand column for comparison.

• represents one infant.

Posture

	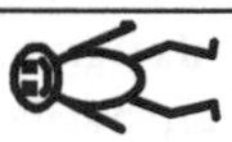 1	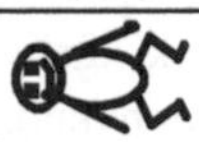 2	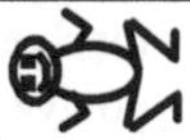 3	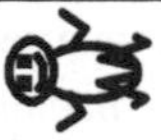 4	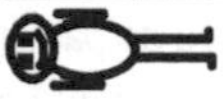 5
day 1		•	• • • • • • • •	• •	
day 5		• •	• •	• • • • • • • • • • • • • • • • • •	

Arm traction

	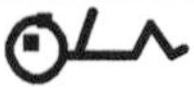	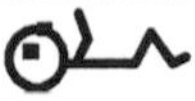	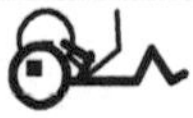	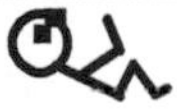	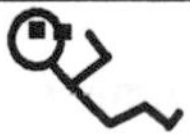
day 1		•	• • • • • • • •	• • • • • • • • • • • • •	• • • • •
day 5	• • • • • • • •	• • • • • • • • • • • • • • • • • • •	• • • • •	• • • • • •	• •

Ventral suspension

	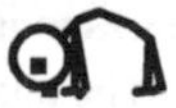	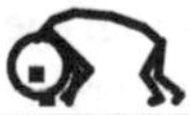	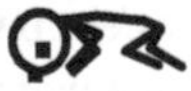	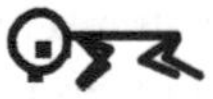	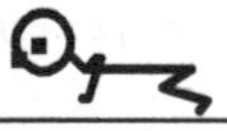
day 1	•	• • • • • •	• •	• • • • • • • • • •	
day 5	•	• • • •	• •	• • • • • • • •	

Moro response

	no response or opening of hands only	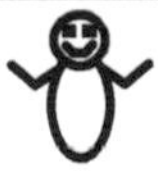	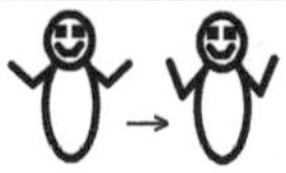 →	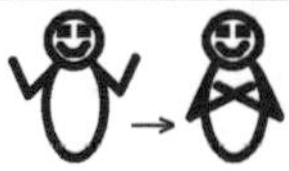 →	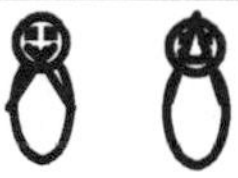 or
day 1			• •	• • • • • • • • • • • • • • •	• •
day 5				• •	• • • • • • • •

Visual alertness

	does not follow or focus on stimuli		stills, focuses, follows briefly to the side but loses stimuli		follows horizontally and vertically; no head turn		follows horizontally and vertically; turns head		follows in a circle	
	B	T	B	T	B	T	B	T	B	T
day 1	• • • • • • • • •		• • • • • •		• • • • • • • • • • • • • • •		• • • • • • • • • •			
day 5	• • •		• • •		• • • • • •		• •		• • •	

Fig. 4.12. Comparison of findings on neurological tests in term infants examined on postnatal days 1 and 5. • represents one infant. B, ball; T, target.

only. Many of the infants were also irritable, but those whose condition remained stable could be pacified. This state persisted for about a week, after which they gradually normalized. If the infant had polycythaemia or hypoglycaemia or hypothermia, the state of hypertonicity would suddenly disappear, often being replaced by hypotonia. The jitteriness ceased and the infant often became less alert and even apathetic. A similar pattern was also seen soon after birth in SGA infants with birth asphyxia. At follow-up, such infants who remained hypertonic were less likely to show abnormal signs during the first year of life than those who became hypotonic. It would thus appear that the hypertonic, hyperexcitable state is optimal for the SGA infant and could indicate an adequate response to stress.

Comment
By observing the neurological system in this sequential way, we have been able (1) to map out the normal process of intrauterine maturation of individual signs in newborn infants of increasing gestational age; (2) to follow the postnatal maturation of preterm infants through to 40 weeks postmenstrual age and beyond; (3) to compare preterm infants of various gestational ages reaching a postnatal age equivalent to 40 weeks postmenstrual age both with each other and with newborn infants of 40 weeks gestation; (4) to establish that in normal preterm infants reaching 40 weeks posmenstrual age, certain responses are *different* from those of newborn term infants and that these differences have to be taken into account in any evaluation; (5) to compare the postnatal maturational process of early preterm infants at other postmenstrual ages, e.g. 36 weeks; and (6) to do longitudinal studies of individual infants in order to identify deviations in the pattern of particular neurological signs under certain pathological circumstances.

5
THE TERM INFANT: DEVELOPMENT OF AN OPTIMALITY SCORE

One criticism of the current method of assessing the neurological status of newborn infants, described in Chapter 3, has been that it does not provide a quantitative scoring system. The method was developed with the primary aim that inspections of the chart should provide easily identifiable patterns that could be correlated with lesions on imaging. Another aim was that variations could be easily recorded on the chart by circling more than one diagram or altering the stick figures. These requirements make it difficult to achieve a quantitative scoring system. However, we also felt that, particularly in a research setting, some quantifications might be useful so that the severity of the neurological findings might be correlated with various insults and the extent of the lesions, particularly in the term infant. To achieve this end, we have developed an optimality scoring system, although for this purpose the recording of the variations could not be scored.

There are a few studies that have already tried to provide a quantitative score for term infants, but in these the definition of abnormality was based on empirical observations rather than on a study of the distributions of patterns in a normal population. In this chapter, we report the results of a study on a normal population of low-risk, term newborn infants born at 37 to 42 weeks gestation. The aim of the study was to evaluate the distribution of the findings for each individual item and their possible variation with gestational age in the range of term birth and to develop an optimality score to help identify possible abnormalities occurring in only a small minority of normal infants (less than 5%).

The revised version of the neurological assessment (see Fig. 2.4) was performed on 250 infants whose parents had volunteered for the project. The only inclusion criteria were (a) that the infants were regarded as normal at birth and sent to the postnatal ward and (b) that their postnatal age was between 6 and 48 hours. As the aim of this study was to assess low-risk, term newborn infants, 26 of the 250 infants were eventually excluded because their gestational age was below 37 weeks or they had shown signs of birth asphyxia, such as an abnormal Apgar score (below 5 at 1 minute and below 7 at 5 minutes) or low cord-blood pH (below 7.2). Thus the optimality score was developed on the basis of the remaining 224 infants.

Calculating optimality scores
OPTIMALITY SCORE FOR INDIVIDUAL ITEMS
The distribution of the raw scores – the grade, or column circled – for the whole population was plotted for each individual item listed on the proforma. The 5th and 10th centiles were taken as cut-off points. The raw score for each item was converted to an optimality score of

1 *(optimal)*, 0.5 *(borderline)*, or 0 *(suboptimal)*, depending on whether the raw score fell, respectively, above the 10th centile, between the 5th and 10th centiles, or below the 5th centile.

The *total optimality score* for an infant was arrived at by summing that infant's optimality scores for all the individual items. This total can range from 0, if all the individual items are suboptimal (below the 5th centile), to a maximum of 34, if all the items are optimal (above the 10th centile). On the basis of the distribution of all these total optimality scores in the population studied, an infant's total optimality score was also classified as optimal, borderline, or suboptimal.

COMPOUND OPTIMALITY SCORE FOR EACH CATEGORY
If more detailed information on individual categories of the examination (tone, tone patterns, reflexes, movements, deviant signs, and orientation and behaviour) is required, a *compound optimality score* for each category can be similarly obtained, by summing the optimality scores for the individual items in the category. The resulting compound optimality score in each category can range from 0 (if every item in the category is suboptimal) to a maximum given by multiplying the highest optimality score obtainable in each item (that is, 1) by the number of items in the category.

RESULTS
The strips from the proforma are shown as reminders of the possible grading of the individual items. For the items that did not vary with gestational age, the exact percentages and conversion to optimality scores are given below the scoring strips. For the items that varied significantly with gestational age, tables showing the evolution of the pattern with gestational age are given.

1) Tone and posture
The raw scores (the number of the column circled) for all items assessing tone, except arm traction, were found to be gestational-age-dependent, showing an increased response from 37 to 42 weeks. The raw score for each item assessing tone was converted to an optimality score, as shown in Table 5.1 (page 93). (Note that the optimality scores depend on the gestational age of the infant.)

POSTURE

1	2	3	4	5
arms & legs extended or very slightly flexed	Legs slightly flexed	legs well flexed but not adducted	legs well flexed & adducted near abdomen	abnormal posture: a) opisthotonus b) marked leg extension, strong arm flexion

Well flexed and adducted legs (column 3 to 4) were found in more than 90% of the infants assessed. The scores for this item were gestational-age-dependent, with limb flexion increasing from 37 to 42 weeks gestation (Fig. 5.1).

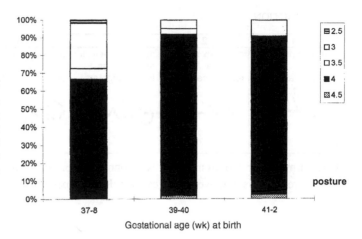

Fig. 5.1. Distribution of raw scores for posture in 224 newborn infants, according to their gestational age at birth. Half points represent responses between two columns (two columns circled on proforma).

ARM RECOIL

1	2	3	4	5
arms do not flex	arms flex slowly, not always; not completely	arms flex slowly; more completely	arms flex quickly and completely	arms difficult to extend; snap back forcefully

Complete recoil (column 3 to 4) was found in more than 90% of the infants assessed. The scores for this item were gestational-age-dependent, with the degree of flexion of the arms increasing from 37 to 42 weeks' gestation (Fig. 5.2).

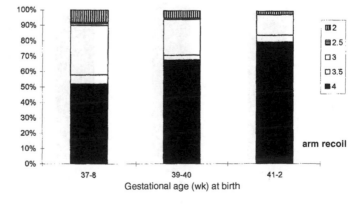

Fig. 5.2. Distribution of raw scores for arm recoil in 224 newborn infants, according to their gestational age at birth.

ARM TRACTION

1	2	3	4	5
arms remain straight; no resistance felt	arms flex slightly or some resistance felt	arms flex well till shoulder lifts, then straighten	arms flex at approx 100° & maintained as shoulder lifts	flexion of arms <100°; maintained when body lifts up

Good arm flexion (column 3 to 4) was found in more than 90% of the infants assessed. The scores for this item were not gestational-age-dependent.

LEG RECOIL

1	2	3	4	5
No flexion	incomplete or variable flexion	complete but slow flexion	complete fast flexion	legs difficult to extend; snap back forcefully

Complete recoil (column 3 to 4) was found in more than 90% of the infants assessed. The scores for this item were gestational-age-dependent (Fig. 5.3).

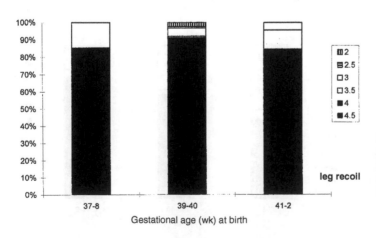

Legend: ▥ 2 ▤ 2.5 ☐ 3 ☐ 3.5 ■ 4 ■ 4.5

leg recoil

Gestational age (wk) at birth

Fig. 5.3. Distribution of raw scores for leg recoil in 224 newborn infants, according to their gestational age at birth.

LEG TRACTION

1	2	3	4	5
legs straight - no resistance felt	legs flex slightly or some resistance felt	legs flex well till bottom lifts up	knee flexes remains flexed when bottom up	flexion stays when back+bottom up

Good leg flexion (column 3 to 4) was found in more than 90% of the infants assessed. The scores for this item were gestational-age-dependent (Fig. 5.4).

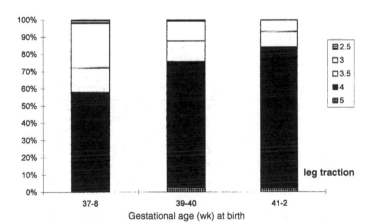

Fig. 5.4. Distribution of raw scores on the leg traction test in 224 newborn infants, according to their gestational age at birth.

POPLITEAL ANGLE

1	2	3	4	5
180°	≈ 150°	≈110°	≈90°	<90°

A popliteal angle between 90° and 110° (column 3 to 4) was found in more than 90% of the infants assessed. The scores for this item were gestational-age-dependent (Fig. 5.5).

89

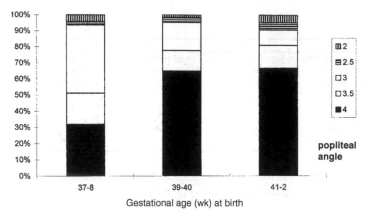

Fig. 5.5. Distribution of raw scores for popliteal angle in 224 newborn infants, according to their gestational age at birth.

popliteal angle

Gestational age (wk) at birth

HEAD CONTROL (1) (EXTENSOR TONE)

1	2	3	4	5
no attempt to raise head	infant tries: effort better felt than seen	raises head but drops forward or back	raises head: remains vertical; it may wobble	

Good head extensor tone (column 3 to 4) was found in more than 90% of the infants assessed. The scores for this item were gestational-age-dependent (Fig. 5.6).

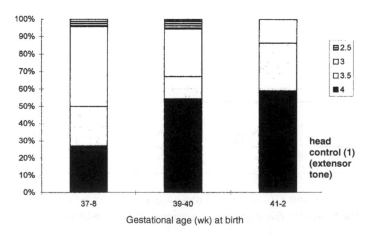

Fig. 5.6. Distribution of raw scores for head control (1) in 224 newborn infants, according to their gestational age at birth.

head control (1) (extensor tone)

Gestational age (wk) at birth

HEAD CONTROL (2) (FLEXOR TONE)

1	2	3	4	5
no attempt to raise head	infant tries: effort better felt than seen	raises head but drops forward or back	raises head: remains vertical; it may wobble	head upright or extended; cannot be passively flexed

Good head flexor tone (column 3 to 4) was found in more than 90% of the infants assessed. The scores for this item were gestational-age-dependent (Fig. 5.7).

Fig. 5.7. Distribution of raw scores for head control (2) in 224 new-born infants, according to their gestational age at birth.

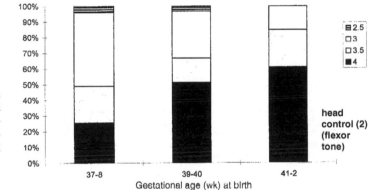

HEAD LAG

1	2	3	4	5
head drops & stays back	tries to lift head but it drops back	able to lift head slightly	lifts head in line with body	head in front of body

When pulled to sit, more than 90% of the infants assessed could lift their head slightly or maintain it in line with their body (column 3 to 4). The scores for this item were gestational-age-dependent (Fig. 5.8).

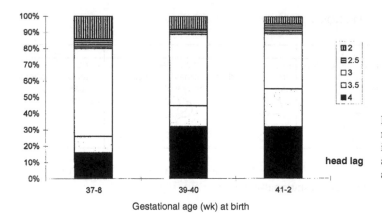

Fig. 5.8. Distribution of raw scores for head lag in 224 newborn infants, according to gestational age at birth.

head lag

Gestational age (wk) at birth

VENTRAL SUSPENSION

1	2	3	4	5
back curved, head & limbs hang straight	back curved, head ↓, limbs slightly flexed	back slightly curved, limbs flexed	back straight, head in line, limbs flexed	back straight, head above body

A slightly curved or extended back (column 3 to 4) was found in more than 90% of the infants assessed. The scores for this item were gestational-age-dependent (Fig. 5.9)

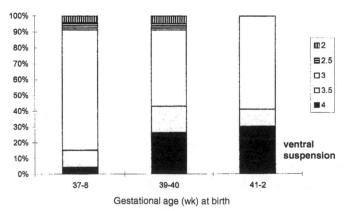

Fig. 5.9. Distribution of raw scores on the ventral suspension test in 224 newborn infants, according to gestational age at birth.

ventral suspension

Gestational age (wk) at birth

TABLE 5.1
Tone items: conversion of newborn infants' raw scores[a] (in body of table) to optimality scores[b] according to gestational age (GA) at birth

	GA 37–38 wk			GA 39–40 wk			GA 41–42 wk		
Optimality score[b]	*1*	*0.5*	*0*	*1*	*0.5*	*0*	*1*	*0.5*	*0*
Posture	4		<3	4	3.5	<3	4	3.5	<3.5
	3		5	3		5			5
Arm recoil	4	2.5	<2.5	4	2.5	<2.5	4		>3
	3		5	3		5	3		5
Arm traction	4		<3	4		<3	4		<3
	3		5	3		5	3		5
Leg recoil	4		<3	4		<3	4		<3
	3		5		3	5	3.5		5
Leg traction	4		<3	4		<3	4	3	<3
	3		5	3		5	3.5		5
Popliteal angle	4	2.5	<2	4		<3	4	2.5	<2.5
	3	2	5	3		5	3		5
Head control (1)	4		<3	4		<3	4		<3
	3		5	3		5	3		5
Head control (2)	4		<3	4		<3	4		<3
	3		5	3		5	3		5
Head lag	4		<2	4	2	<2	4	2.5	<2.5
	3		5	3		5	3		5
	2			2.5					
Ventral suspension	4	2.5	<2.5	4	2.5	<2.5	4		<3
	3		5	3		5	3		5

[a] Raw score: column circled on proforma.
[b] Optimality score:
  1 optimal (in bold type): >10th centile; raw score found in 90% of population or more
  0.5 borderline: between 5th and 10th centiles; raw score found in more than 5% but less than 10%
  0 suboptimal: <5th centile; raw score found in less than 5%.

COMPOUND OPTIMALITY SCORE FOR TONE ITEMS

The optimality scores for the 10 individual items assessing tone were summed to obtain a compound optimality score for tone. In this category, the compound optimality score can range from 0 (all items suboptimal) to 10 (all 10 items optimal).

In our cohort, the compound optimality scores for tone ranged from 4.5 to 10. Scores of 9 or more were found in 95% of the infants assessed and were classed as optimal. Scores below 9 (<5th centile) were suboptimal.

2) Tone patterns

This section of the examination assesses patterns of limb tone and head control by comparing the raw scores for certain individual items assessing tone. The raw score for each of these items was converted to an optimality score, as shown in Table 5.2 (page 95).

FLEXOR TONE (1) (ON TRACTION: ARMS VERSUS LEGS)

1	2	3	4	5
	score for arm flexion less than leg flexion	score for arm flexion equal to leg flexion	score for arm flexion more than leg flexion but difference 1 column or less	score for arm flexion more than leg flexion but difference more than 1 column
	25%	63%	12%	<1%

incidence

The optimal patterns were arm flexion less than or equal to leg flexion on the respective traction tests (column 2 or 3, respectively), or greater than leg flexion by one column or less (column 4). Arm flexion greater than leg flexion by more than one column was classed as suboptimal.

FLEXOR TONE (2) (IN SUPINE INFANT: ARMS VERSUS LEGS)

1	2	3	4	5
		arms and legs flexed	strong arm flexion with strong leg extension *intermittent*	strong arm flexion with strong leg extension *continuous*
		100	<1%	<1%

incidence

The optimal pattern in the supine infant was equal arm and leg flexion (column 3). Both other patterns were classed as suboptimal.

LEG EXTENSOR TONE

1	2	3	4	5
	score for leg traction more than score for popliteal angle	score for leg traction equal to score for popliteal angle	score for leg traction less than score for popliteal angle, by 1 column only	score for leg traction less than score for popliteal angle, by more than 1 column
	4%	57%	35%	1%

incidence

A raw score for popliteal angle equal to that on the leg traction test (column 3) or more than that on the leg traction test by one column or less (column 4) was classed as optimal; both other patterns were classed as suboptimal.

HEAD CONTROL IN FLEXION AND EXTENSION

1	2	3	4	5
	score for head extension less than head flexion	score for head extension equal to head flexion	score for head extension more than head flexion, but difference 1 column or less	score for head extension more than head flexion but difference more than 1 column
	3%	94%	3%	<1%

incidence

Head extension equal to head flexion (column 3) was found in 94% of our cohort and was classed as optimal; all the other patterns were classed as suboptimal.

94

1	2	3	4	5
	score for ventral suspension less than head lag	score for ventral suspension equal to head lag	score for ventral suspension more than head lag but difference 1 column or less	score for ventral suspension more than head lag but difference more than 1 column
	24%	55%	16%	<1%

Incidence

A ventral suspension score less than or the same as that for head lag (column 2 or 3 circled for this item), equal to that for head lag (column 3), or greater by one column or less (column 4) was classed as optimal. A score for ventral suspension greater than that for head lag by more than one column was classed as suboptimal.

TABLE 5.2

Tone patterns: conversion of newborn infants' raw scores[a] (in body of table) to optimality scores[b]

	Optimality score[b]		
	1	*0.5*	*0*
	Raw score[a]		
Flexor tone (1)	4		5
on traction (arms versus legs)	3		
	2		
Flexor tone (2)	3		4
in supine infant (arms versus legs)			5
Leg extensor tone	4		<3
	3		5
Head control (1) and (2)	3		<3
			4
			5
Head lag and ventral suspension	4		5
	3		
	2		

[a] Raw score: column circled on proforma.

[b] Optimality score:

1 optimal (in bold type): >10th centile; raw score found in 90% of population or more

0.5 borderline: between 5th and 10th centiles; raw score found in more than 5% but less than 10%

0 suboptimal: <5th centile; raw score found in less than 5%.

COMPOUND OPTIMALITY SCORES FOR TONE PATTERNS

The optimality scores for the individual items assessing tone pattern were summed to obtain a compound optimality score for tone patterns.

In this category, the compound optimality score could range from 0 (all items suboptimal) to 5 (all five items optimal). As the compound optimality score was 5 in all the infants assessed, scores of 5 were classed as optimal, and below 5 as suboptimal.

3) Movements

None of the raw scores for items assessing movements was age-dependent. The results for each individual item are summarized below. The raw score for each item assessing movement was converted to an optimality score, as shown in Table 5.3.

SPONTANEOUS MOVEMENT (QUANTITY)

1	2	3	4	5
no movement	sporadic and short isolated movements	frequent isolated movements	frequent generalized movements	continuous exaggerated movements
<1	3%	5%	92%	<1%

incidence

Frequent generalized alternating movements (column 4) were classed as optimal. Frequent isolated movements (column 3) were classed as borderline, and all the other patterns as suboptimal.

SPONTANEOUS MOVEMENT (QUALITY)

1	2	3	4	5
only stretches	stretches and random abrupt movements; some smooth movements	fluent movements but monotonous	fluent alternating movements of arms + legs; good variability	• cramped, synchronized; • mouthing • jerky or other abnormal movements
2	5%	<1%	93%	<1%

incidence

Fluent alternating movements (column 4) with good variability were classed as optimal. Frequent stretches alternating with fluent, smooth movements (column 2) were classed as borderline, and all the other patterns as suboptimal.

HEAD RAISING PRONE

1	2	3	4	5
no response	infant rolls head over, chin not raised	infant raises chin, rolls head over	infant brings head and chin up	infant brings head up and keeps it up
<1	10%	50%	40%	<1%

incidence

When infants were put in the prone position, raising the chin and rolling the head over (column 3) or bringing the whole head up (column 4) was classed as optimal. Rolling the head over without raising the chin (column 2) was classed as borderline, and all the other responses as suboptimal.

TABLE 5.3
Spontaneous movement: conversion of newborn infants' raw
scores[a] (in body of table) to optimality scores[b]

	Optimality score[b]		
	1	0.5	0
	Raw score[a]		
Movement (quantity)	**4**	3	<3 5
Movement (quality)	**4**	3	<3 5
Head raising	**4** **3**		<3
37/38 weeks only		2.5	<2.5

[a] Raw score: column circled on proforma.
[b] Optimality score:
  1 optimal (in bold type): >10th centile; raw score found in 90% of population or more
  0.5 borderline: between 5th and 10th centiles; raw score found in more than 5% but less than 10%
  0 suboptimal: <5th centile; raw score found in less than 5%.

COMPOUND OPTIMALITY SCORE FOR MOVEMENTS
The optimality scores for individual items were summed to obtain a compound optimality score for movements. In this category, the compound optimality score could range from 0 (all items suboptimal) to 3 (all three items optimal).

In our cohort, the compound optimality score ranged from 1 to 3. A score of 3 was found in more than 96% of the infants assessed and was classed as optimal. Scores below 3 were classed as suboptimal.

4) Reflexes
None of the reflexes was age-dependent except the Moro reflex. The results for each individual item are summarized below. The raw score for each item assesssing reflexes was converted to an optimality score, as shown in Table 5.4 (page 99).

TENDON REFLEXES

1	2	3	4	5
absent	felt, not seen	seen	"exaggerated" (very brisk)	clonus
<1	21%	78%	<1%	<1%

incidence

Reflexes that were easily elicitable (column 3) or that could be felt but not seen (column 2) were classed as optimal, and all the other responses as suboptimal.

SUCK/GAG REFLEX

1	2	3	4	5
no gag / no suck	weak irregular suck only No stripping	weak regular suck Some stripping	strong suck: (a) irregular (b) regular Good stripping	no suck but strong clenching
0	1%	5%	92%	2%

incidence

A strong suck (column 3) was classed as optimal, a weak suck (column 2) as borderline, and all the other responses as suboptimal.

PALMAR GRASP

1	2	3	4	5
	short, weak flexion of fingers	strong flexion of fingers	strong finger flexion, shoulder ↑	very strong grasp; infant can be lifted off couch
<1%	6%	85%	9%	<1%

incidence

Strong flexion of the fingers (column 3) was classed as optimal. Short, weak flexion of the fingers and strong flexion with lifting of the shoulder (scores of 2 and 4) were classed as borderline and all the other responses as suboptimal.

PLANTAR GRASP

1	2	3	4	5
no response	partial plantar flexion of toes	toes curve around the examiner's finger		
<1%	2%	98%		

incidence

A strong plantar grasp with toes curving around the examiner's finger (column 3) was classed as optimal and all the other responses as suboptimal.

MORO REFLEX

1	2	3	4	5
no response, or opening of hands only	full abduction at shoulder and extension of the arms; no adduction	full abduction, but only delayed or partial adduction	partial abduction at shoulder, and extension of arms followed by smooth adduction	• minimal abduction or adduction • no abduction or adduction; only forward extension of arms • marked adduction only

Partial or full abduction with partial or full adduction (column 3 to 4) was found in more than 90% of the infants assessed. The scores for this item were gestational-age-dependent.

In infants born at 37 to 38 weeks, a response in column 3 to 4 was optimal, whereas the only optimal response in term infants born later than 38 weeks was column 4. See Table 5.4 for other variations in these optimality scores.

PLACING

1	2	3	4	5
no response	dorsiflexion of ankle only	full placing response with flexion of hip and knee & placing sole on surface		
1%	18%	81% Incidence		

A full placing response with flexion of hip, knee, and ankle (column 3) or flexion of the ankle only (column 2) was classed as optimal and the absence of response as suboptimal.

TABLE 5.4
Reflexes: conversion of newborn infants' raw scores[a] (in body of table) to optimality scores[b]

	Optimality score[b]		
	1	*0.5*	*0*
	Raw score[a]		
Tendon reflex	**3** **2**		<2 4 5
Sucking reflex	**3**	2	<2 4 5
Palmar grasp	**4** **3**	2	<2 5
Plantar grasp	**3**		<3 5
Placing reflex	**3** **2**		<2 5

	GA 37–38 wk			GA 39–40 wk			GA 41–42 wk		
Optimality score[b]	*1*	*0.5*	*0*	*1*	*0.5*	*0*	*1*	*0.5*	*0*
Moro reflex[c]	**4** **3**		<3 5	**4**	3.5 3	<3 5	**4**	3.5	<3.5 5

[a] Raw score: column circled on proforma.
[b] Optimality score:
  1   optimal (in bold type): >10th centile; raw score found in 90% of population or more
  0.5 borderline: between 5th and 10th centiles; raw score found in more than 5% but less than 10%
  0   suboptimal: <5th centile; raw score found in less than 5%.
[c] According to gestational age (GA) at birth.

COMPOUND OPTIMALITY SCORE FOR REFLEXES

The optimality scores for individual items were summed to obtain a compound optimality score for reflexes. In this category, the compound optimality score could range from 0 (all items suboptimal) to 6 (all 6 items optimal).

In our cohort, the compound optimality score ranged from 4 to 6. Scores of 5 or above were found in 97% of the infants assessed and were classed as optimal. Scores below 5 were classed as suboptimal.

5) Abnormal signs

None of the raw scores for abnormal signs was age-dependent. The results for each individual item are summarized below. The raw score for each item assessing abnormal signs was converted to an optimality score, as shown in Table 5.5.

ABNORMAL HAND OR TOE POSTURE

1	2	3	4	5
	hands open, toes straight most of the time	intermittent fisting or thumb adduction	continuous fisting or thumb adduction; index finger flexion, thumb opposition	continuous big toe extension or flexion of all toes
	85%	12% Incidence	3%	<1%

Hands open and normal posture of the toes (column 2) and intermittent hand fisting or adduction of thumb (column 3) were classed as optimal and both other patterns as suboptimal.

TREMORS

1	2	3	4	5
	no tremor, or tremor only when crying or only after Moro reflex	tremor occasionally when awake	frequent tremors when awake	continuous tremors
	88%	12% Incidence	<1%	<1%

No tremor (or tremors only when crying) (column 2), or tremor only after a Moro reflex or occasionally when awake (column 3) were classed as optimal and both other patterns as suboptimal.

STARTLES

1	2	3	4	5
no startle even to sudden noise	no spontaneous startle but reacts to sudden noise	2-3 spontaneous startles	more than 3 spontaneous startles	continuous startles
<1%	94%	6% Incidence	<1%	<1%

Absence of spontaneous startles (column 2) was classed as optimal, or two or three spontaneous startles (column 3) as borderline, and all the other patterns as suboptimal.

TABLE 5.5
**Abnormal signs: conversion of newborn infants' raw
scores[a] (in body of table) to optimality scores[b]**

	Optimality score[b]		
	1	*0.5*	*0*
	Raw score[a]		
Hand or toe posture	**3**		1
	2		>3
Tremors	**3**		1
	2		>3
Startles	**2**	3	1
			>3

[a] Raw score: column circled on proforma.

[b] Optimality score:

1 optimal (in bold type): >10th centile; raw score found in
   90% of population or more

0.5 borderline: between 5th and 10th centiles; raw score found
   in more than 5% but less than 10%

0 suboptimal: <5th centile; raw score found in less than 5%.

COMPOUND OPTIMALITY SCORE FOR ABNORMAL SIGNS

The optimality scores for individual items were summed to obtain a compound optimality
score for abnormal signs. In this category, the compound optimality score could range from
0 (all items suboptimal) to 3 (all 3 items optimal).

In our cohort, the compound optimality score ranged from 1 to 3. A score of 3 was found
in 97% of the infants assessed and was classed as optimal. Scores below 3 were classed as
suboptimal.

6) Orientation and behaviour

None of the items assessing behaviour was age-dependent. The results for each individual
item are summarized below. The raw score for each item assessing orientation and behaviour was converted to an optimality score, as shown in Table 5.6 (page 103).

EYE MOVEMENTS

1	2	3	4	5
does not open eyes		full conjugated eye movements	*transient* • nystagmus • strabismus • roving eye movements • sunset sign	*persistent* • nystagmus • strabismus • roving eye movements abnormal pupils
7%		92% **Incidence**	1%	<1%

Opening of the eyes could not be obtained in 7% (column 1). Normal symmetrical eye movements (column 3) were classed as optimal and both the other patterns as suboptimal.

AUDITORY ORIENTATION

1	2	3	4	5
no reaction	auditory startle; brightens and stills; no true orientation	shifting of eyes, head might turn towards source	prolonged head turn to stimulus; search with eyes; smooth	turns head (jerkily, abruptly) & eyes towards noise every time
<1%	30%	50% **incidence**	20%	<1%

Eye and head turning towards the side of the noise (column 3 to 4) or a weaker response (brightening) (column 2) were classed as optimal and both other responses as suboptimal.

VISUAL ORIENTATION

1		2		3		4		5	
does not follow or focus on stimuli		stills, focuses, follows briefly to the side but loses stimuli		follows horizontally and vertically; no head turn		follows horizontally and vertically; turns head		follows in a circle	
B	T	B	T	B	T	B	T	B	T
<1%		7%		41% **incidence**		51%		1%	

In 7% of the infants, the eyes remained closed throughout the examination and visual orientation could not be tested (not shown in scoring strip). In the remaining infants, the ability to track horizontally and vertically, with or without head movements (column 3 to 4) was classed as optimal. Incomplete tracking (column 2) was classed as borderline and both other responses as suboptimal.

ALERTNESS

1	2	3	4	5
will not respond to stimuli	when awake, looks only briefly	when awake, looks at stimuli but loses them	keeps interest in stimuli	does not tire (hyper-reactive)
1%	2%	38% **incidence**	49%	<1%

This was tested as the quality of the infant's response to track the stimulus presented (a red ball or a target). Looking at the stimulus briefly (column 3) or at length (column 4) was classed as optimal and all the other responses as suboptimal.

IRRITABILITY

1	2	3	4	5
quiet all the time, not irritable to any stimuli	awakes, cries sometimes when handled	cries often when handled	cries always when handled	cries even when not handled
<1%	93%	5% **incidence**	2%	<1%

Occasional crying when handled (column 2) was classed as optimal. Frequent crying when handled (column 3) was classed as borderline and all the other patterns as suboptimal.

CONSOLABILITY

1	2	3	4	5
not crying; consoling not needed	cries briefly; consoling not needed	cries; becomes quiet when talked to	cries; needs picking up to be consoled	cries; cannot be consoled
1%	41%	45%	12%	<1%

incidence

Infants who did not cry or who cried briefly but either did not need consoling or could be consoled by talking or by being picked up (scores of 2, 3, or 4) were classed as optimal. Both the other patterns were classed as suboptimal.

CRY

1	2	3	4	5
no cry at all	whimpering cry only	cries to stimuli but normal pitch		High-pitched cry; often continuous
<!%	7%	92%		1%

incidence

A normal cry in response to stimuli (column 3) was classed as optimal. A whimpering cry (column 2) was classed as borderline and both other responses as suboptimal.

TABLE 5.6
Behaviour: conversion of newborn infants' raw scores[a] (in body of table) to optimality scores[b]

	Optimality score[b]		
	1	*0.5*	*0*
	Raw score[a]		
Eyes	**3**	1	2
			>3
Auditory orientation	**4**		<2
	3		5
	2		
Visual orientation	**4**		<3
	3		5
Alertness	**4**		<3
	3		5
Irritability	**2**	3	1
			>3
Consolability	**4**		<2
	3		5
	2		
Cry	**3**	2	1
			5

[a] Raw score: column circled on proforma.
[b] Optimality score:
  1   optimal (in bold type): >10th centile; raw score found in 90% of population or more
  0.5 borderline: between 5th and 10th centiles; raw score found in more than 5% but less than 10%
  0   suboptimal: <5th centile; raw score found in less than 5%.

The optimality scores for individual items were summed to obtain a compound optimality score for behaviour. In this category, the compound optimality score could range from 0 (all items suboptimal) to 7 (all 7 items optimal).In our cohort, the compound optimality score for orientation and behaviour ranged from 5 to 7. Scores of 6 or more were found in 96% of the infants assessed and were classed as optimal. All scores below 6 were classed as suboptimal.

Total neurological optimality score

The total optimality score for each infant, obtained by summing the infant's optimality scores on all 34 items in the whole examination, ranged from 25 to 34. More than 95% of the infants assessed had scores between 30.5 and 34, and these scores were classed as optimal. Scores below 30.5 were classed as suboptimal.

Comments

Using the cut-off points of the 10th and 5th centiles for each item, we classed as optimal not only the most frequently observed pattern, but also other patterns that, though not as common, were observed in more than 10% of our normal population born at term (37 to 42 weeks).

We found that variations with gestational age may occur even in infants who were born at term, and these changes have to be taken in account in defining an optimality score. While the items assessing orientation and behaviour and those assessing alertness showed little variation with gestational age, others showed a consistent variation between 37 and 42 weeks.

In our cohort, an optimality score of less than 31/34 was found in fewer than 10%, while deviant scores on one or two single items were achieved in a third of the normal population, suggesting that isolated deviant signs have little diagnostic value.

Even a suboptimal global score, however, does not necessarily indicate that the infant is neurologically abnormal, but indicates only that the infant needs to be reassessed. Serial examination will allow one to differentiate the infants who show persistent abnormalities, and thus need further investigations, from the ones with transient signs related to temporary causes such as maternal anaesthesia, analgesia, or hypoglycaemia.

In conclusion, although at present this approach may still be too complex for routine clinical use, it has the advantage that, in research settings, more quantitative and detailed information of the neurological status of the infants in the first days of life can be achieved. The introduction of the optimality score allows comparison of clinical findings with neurophysiological and imaging findings, and should increase its potential use in longitudinal follow-up studies.

6
THE NEUROLOGICAL EXAMINATION IN PRETERM AND TERM INFANTS WITH BRAIN LESIONS

The method of neurological assessment described in this book has proved useful in diagnosing and following the evolution of certain pathological conditions. In particular, using the method in combination with imaging and neurophysiological techniques has made it possible to specify more clearly than hitherto the clinical patterns associated with various brain lesions. Our main experience has been with periventricular leukomalacia and haemorrhages in preterm infants and in focal infarction and hypoxic–ischaemic encephalopathy (HIE) in term infants.

Germinal matrix haemorrhage and intraventricular haemorrhage
Periventricular/intraventricular haemorrhage (IVH) is the most common brain lesion observed in the neonatal period. It occurs mainly in low-birthweight preterm infants, in whom the incidence has been reported to range from 15 to 40%, depending on gestational age. The classifications of IVH have been mainly based on its location and extent (for reviews see Govaert and de Vries 1997, Rennie 1997). The classification we use (Fig. 6.1) is as follows:
• **Grade I:** localized to the germinal layer.
• **Grade II:** extends into the basal ganglia. This grade can be subdivided according to the quantity of blood in the ventricles: in grade IIa, there is only a small amount of blood in the lateral ventricles, whereas in grade IIb, 50% or more of the ventricular system is filled with blood.
• **Grade III:** the blood in the ventricles is in continuity with blood in the parenchyma.

NEONATAL CLINICAL SIGNS AND THEIR EVOLUTION
Before the introduction of routine brain ultrasonography in the neonatal unit, only the large haemorrhages were clinically recognized. Volpe (1978) described three characteristic syndromes in association with these lesions. One is the clinical presentation he called "catastrophic deterioration syndrome"; this usually occurs in infants who do not survive the haemorrhage. The accompanying signs are stupor, coma, apnoea, generalized tonic seizures, fixed pupils, and flaccid quadriparesis. Volpe speculated that the syndrome reflects a movement of blood through the ventricular system, sequentially affecting the diencephalon, midbrain, pons, and medulla. He described another clinical presentation as the "saltatory syndrome", characterized by alterations in the level of consciousness, changes in the quantity and quality of spontaneous movement, and aberrations of eye position and movement.

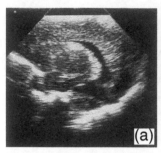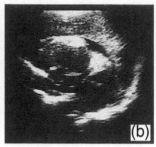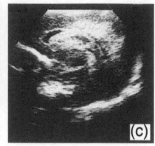

Fig. 6.1. Gradings of haemorrhages on ultrasound in parasagittal view. (a) Grade I – the haemorrhage is localized to the germinal layer; (b) grade II – the haemorrhage is seen in the ventricles and involves the basal ganglia; (c) grade III – there is blood in the ventricle and in the parenchyma.

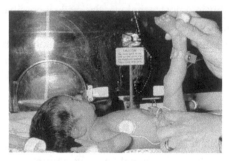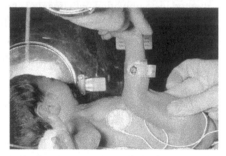

Fig. 6.2. Infant early during IVH. Note that despite the poor tone in the leg on traction, the popliteal angle is only 100°.

Alternating deterioration and improvement continue over many hours. Volpe called a third clinical presentation the "silent syndrome"; this occurs in 25 to 50% of the infants with IVH, in whom the clinical signs are very subtle and can easily be missed.

The advent of cranial ultrasonography and computed tomography has made it possible to correlate clinical findings directly with the site, size, and evolution of these haemorrhagic lesions. By comparing serial ultrasound findings with repeated clinical evaluations, it was possible to identify clinically (Dubowitz et al. 1981) haemorrhages that in the past have been considered silent (Papile et al. 1978) and to map out three distinct clinical stages in infants with germinal matrix/intraventricular haemorrhage (Dubowitz et al. 1981).

- **Stage 1.** Preceding the ultrasound evidence of haemorrhage or at the time of onset, hypertonicity (more marked in the arms) and excessive motility with tremors and startles may be noted. Tendon reflexes are brisk, the Moro reflex is exaggerated, and the infant is usually irritable. There is no visual or auditory orientation.

- **Stage 2** can be seen when there is established haemorrhage. Tone and motility are decreased. One of the most common signs at this stage is that the popliteal angle is small (tight) relative to the leg tone seen on leg traction (Fig. 6.2). Tremors and startles are absent. Reactivity is generally poor. Visual orientation is absent and auditory responses can be variable.

- **Stage 3** is the phase of recovery, usually starting at the end of the first week. Limb tone, including the popliteal angle, becomes normal first. Motility improves next. Then auditory orientation recovers, followed by visual orientation. Head and trunk control are the last to normalize. During this phase, roving eye movements are often observed. In infants who later show abnormal development, a number of deviant signs may be noticeable at this stage. The duration of recovery can be quite variable (see Table 6.1, page 115) and some infants still show tremors and trunk hypotonia even when examined at 40 weeks post-menstrual age. These signs, however, when present, are usually mild. Interestingly, the severity of the early clinical signs does not necessarily relate to the extent of the haemorrhagic lesion or to outcome.

Figures 6.3 and 6.4 show ultrasound findings and outcome in an infant with a large haemorrhage. Figure 6.5 shows the evolution of the neurological examination from postnatal day 1 (Fig. 6.5a), before the haemorrhage could be detected on neonatal ultrasound, to day 5 (Fig. 6.5b), 3 days after the onset of the haemorrhage. Clinical findings and outcome are shown in Figs. 6.6 to 6.11.

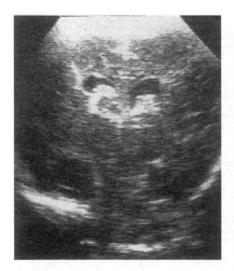 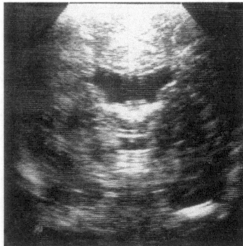

Fig. 6.3. Ultrasound scan made at 20 hours of age in an infant born at 30 weeks gestation. Note the large haemorrhage filling more than 50% of the lateral ventricles.

Fig. 6.4. Ultrasound scan made in the same child at 3 weeks of age. Note the persistent ventricular dilatation.

IVH day 1

POSTURE Infant supine. Look mainly at position of legs but also note arms. *Score predominant posture.*	arms & legs extended or very slightly flexed	Legs slightly flexed	legs well flexed but not adducted	legs well flexed & adducted near abdomen	abnormal posture: a) opisthotonus b) marked leg extension, strong arm flexion		
ARM RECOIL Take both hands, quickly extend arms parallel to the body, Count to three. Release. Repeat 3 times.	arms do not flex	arms flex slowly, not always; not completely	arms flex slowly; more completely	arms flex quickly and completely	arms difficult to extend; snap back forcefully		
ARM TRACTION Hold wrist and pull arm upwards. Note flexion at elbow and resistance while shoulder lifts off table. *Test each side separately.*	arms remain straight; no resistance felt	arms flex slightly or some resistance felt	arms flex well till shoulder lifts, then straighten	arms flex at approx 100° & maintained as shoulder lifts	flexion of arms <100°; maintained when body lifts up		
LEG RECOIL Take *both* ankles in one hand, flex hips + knees. Quickly extend. Release. Repeat 3 times.	No flexion	incomplete or variable flexion	complete but slow flexion	complete fast flexion	legs difficult to extend; snap back forcefully		
LEG TRACTION Grasp ankle and slowly pull leg upwards. Note flexion at knees and resistance as buttocks lift. *Test each side separately.*	legs straight - no resistance felt	legs flex slightly or some resistance felt	legs flex well till bottom lifts up	knee flexes remains flexed when bottom up	flexion stays when back+bottom up		
POPLITEAL ANGLE Fix knee on abdomen, extend leg by gentle pressure with index finger behind the ankle. Note angle at knee. *Test each side separately.*	180°	≈150°	≈110°	≈90°	<90°		
HEAD CONTROL (1) *(extensor tone)* Infant sitting upright. Encircle chest with both hands holding shoulders. Let head drop forward.	no attempt to raise head	infant tries: effort better felt than seen	raises head but drops forward or back	raises head: remains vertical; it may wobble			
HEAD CONTROL (2) *(flexor tone)* Infant sitting upright. Encircle chest with both hands holding shoulders. Let head drop backward.	no attempt to raise head	infant tries: effort better felt than seen	raises head but drops forward or back	raises head: remains vertical; it may wobble	head upright or extended; cannot be passively flexed		
HEAD LAG Pull infant towards sitting posture by traction on both wrists & support head slightly. Also note arm flexion.	head drops & stays back	tries to lift head but it drops back	able to lift head slightly	lifts head in line with body	head in front of body		
VENTRAL SUSPENSION Hold infant in ventral suspension. Observe back, flexion of limbs, and relation of head to trunk. If it looks different, DRAW.	back curved, head & limbs hang straight	back curved, head ↓, limbs slightly flexed	back slightly curved, limbs flexed	back straight, head in line, limbs flexed	back straight, head above body		

Fig. 6.5a. Findings on neurological examination of an infant who had an intraventricular haemorrhage on postnatal day 4. The examinations were on day 1 (a; above) and day 5 (b; facing page) (before and after the haemorrhage, respectively).

IVH day 5

POSTURE Infant supine. Look mainly at position of legs but also note arms. *Score predominant posture.*	arms & legs extended or very slightly flexed	legs slightly flexed	legs well flexed but not adducted	legs well flexed & adducted near abdomen	abnormal posture: a) opisthotonus b) marked leg extension, strong arm flexion		
ARM RECOIL Take both hands, quickly extend arms parallel to the body, Count to three. Release. Repeat 3 times.	arms do not flex	arms flex slowly, not always; not completely	arms flex slowly; more completely	arms flex quickly and completely	arms difficult to extend; snap back forcefully		
ARM TRACTION Hold wrist and pull arm upwards. Note flexion at elbow and resistance while shoulder lifts off table. *Test each side separately.* R L	arms remain straight; no resistance felt R L	arms flex slightly or some resistance felt R L	arms flex well till shoulder lifts, then straighten R L	arms flex at approx 100° & maintained as shoulder lifts R L	flexion of arms <100°; maintained when body lifts up R L		
LEG RECOIL Take *both* ankles in one hand, flex hips + knees. Quickly extend. Release. Repeat 3 times.	No flexion	incomplete or variable flexion	complete but slow flexion	complete fast flexion	legs difficult to extend; snap back forcefully		
LEG TRACTION Grasp ankle and slowly pull leg upwards. Note flexion at knees and resistance as buttocks lift. *Test each side separately.* R L	legs straight - no resistance felt R L	legs flex slightly or some resistance felt R L	legs flex well till bottom lifts up R L	knee flexes remains flexed when bottom up R L	flexion stays when back+bottom up R L		
POPLITEAL ANGLE Fix knee on abdomen, extend leg by gentle pressure with index finger behind the ankle. Note angle at knee. *Test each side separately.* R L	180° R L	≈150° R L	≈110° R L	≈90° R L	<90° R L		
HEAD CONTROL (1) *(extensor tone)* Infant sitting upright. Encircle chest with both hands holding shoulders. Let head drop forward.	no attempt to raise head	infant tries: effort better felt than seen	raises head but drops forward or back	raises head: remains vertical; it may wobble			
HEAD CONTROL (2) *(flexor tone)* Infant sitting upright. Encircle chest with both hands holding shoulders. Let head drop backward.	no attempt to raise head	infant tries: effort better felt than seen	raises head but drops forward or back	raises head: remains vertical; it may wobble	head upright or extended; cannot be passively flexed		
HEAD LAG Pull infant towards sitting posture by traction on both wrists & support head slightly. Also note arm flexion.	head drops & stays back	tries to lift head but it drops back	able to lift head slightly	lifts head in line with body	head in front of body		
VENTRAL SUSPENSION Hold infant in ventral suspension. Observe back, flexion of limbs, and relation of head to trunk. If it looks different, DRAW.	back curved, head & limbs hang straight	back curved, head ↓, limbs slightly flexed	back slightly curved, limbs flexed	back straight, head in line, limbs flexed	back straight, head above body		

Fig. 6.5b. Findings of neurological examination on postnatal day 5 of an infant who had had an intraventricular haemorrhage the previous day. Compare prehaemorrhage findings in Figure 6.5a.

109

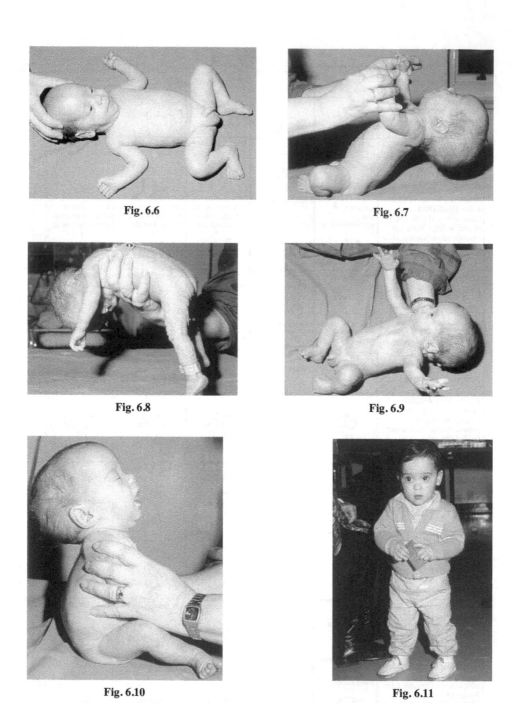

Fig. 6.6

Fig. 6.7

Fig. 6.8

Fig. 6.9

Fig. 6.10

Fig. 6.11

Figs. 6.6–6.11. At 40 weeks postmenstrual age, the infant (same as in Figs. 6.3 and 6.4) had hypotonic posture (6.6), head lag (6.7), and poor ventral suspension (6.8). The Moro reflex consisted mainly of full abduction (6.9). When the infant was held in a sitting position, an increase in neck extensor tone was also noted (6.10). At 18 months, the child was neurologically normal (6.11).

Periventricular leukomalacia

The term *periventricular leukomalacia* was introduced by Banker and Larroche in 1962 to indicate white matter lesions in the periventricular areas in pathological specimens. The advent of ultrasound equipment with high-frequency transducers and of MRI has improved the identification of these lesions in vivo (Figs. 6.12, 6.13).

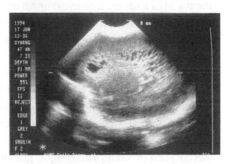

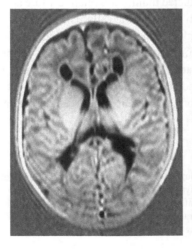

Fig. 6.12. Cranial ultrasound in a female infant born at 29 weeks gestation showing bilateral periventricular changes with cystic degeneration on both coronal and sagittal views.

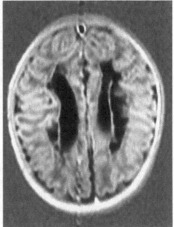

Fig. 6.13. The MRI (inversion recovery) showed mildly dilated but squared ventricles with abnormal signal intensity in the periventricular regions (both images).

111

Several classifications for leukomalacia have been proposed. The one suggested by de Vries et al. (1992) is quite comprehensive and is easy to apply:

- **Grade I:** transient periventricular densities (less than 7 days);
- **Grade II:** localized cysts in the external angle of the lateral ventricle;
- **Grade III:** extensive cysts in frontoparietal and/or occipital periventricular white matter (cystic periventricular leukomalacia);
- **Grade IV:** extensive cysts in subcortical white matter (cystic subcortical leukomalacia).

NEONATAL CLINICAL SIGNS AND THEIR EVOLUTION

Grades I and II leukomalacia are often associated with a normal neurological examination or with only very minor signs. The outcome in children with leukomalacia of these two grades is generally good, although recent studies have suggested that some present with minor neurological signs or perceptual motor difficulties at school age (Jongmans et al. 1993, 1997). Cystic lesions, however, have a more adverse outcome, and some deviant signs can be identified in the first weeks of life.

If the insult occurred some weeks before delivery, during fetal life, the infant might generally show only some degree of hypotonia and mild lethargy at birth. If the lesion is the result of a severe ischaemic insult during the perinatal or neonatal period, clinical signs are generally more prominent, with a more marked initial hypotonia and lethargy; auditory and visual responses are usually age appropriate. The infant then improves and for a period of 4 to 6 weeks may appear near normal (Fig. 6.14–6.21).

Six to 10 weeks after the insult, a very characteristic clinical picture emerges. Infants gradually become more and more irritable, but the cry is of normal pitch. Feeding may be the only way to pacify them. They exhibit a very abnormal tone pattern, with marked increase of flexor tone in the arms and extensor tone in the legs (Fig. 6.22). Marked neck extensor hypertonia is usually present. Movements may be normal but more often are stereotyped or cramped. Tongue protrusion is often present, giving the impression of hypothyroidism. Fisting and adducted thumbs are relatively rare at this stage but abnormal finger and toe postures are usually present bilaterally. The finger posture consists of flexion of the thumb and index finger with the other fingers extended. The big toe is spontaneously dorsiflexed. The placing reaction is poor. The Moro reflex is abnormal, consisting of forward extension only, with hardly any abduction or adduction. Frequent tremors and startles may be noted. Visual and auditory functions are normal at this stage (Fig. 6.23). At first the pattern shows little or no differences between the infants with periventricular and subcortical lesions.

Figs. 6.14–6.21 *(facing page).* Evolution of clinical signs in PVL. Relatively normal posture in the supine position (6.14) and relative hypotonicity (6.15–6.17) at 33 weeks postmenstrual age (2 weeks postnatally). Four weeks later the infant showed an extended posture (6.18); but note that the head control in the pull-to-sit test, on ventral suspension, and while sitting (6.19–6.21) appeared normal (too good for the infant's postmenstrual age).

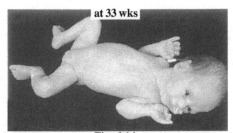

at 33 wks

Fig. 6.14

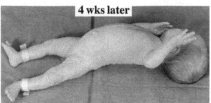

4 wks later

Fig. 6.18

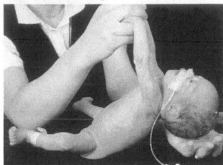

Fig. 6.15

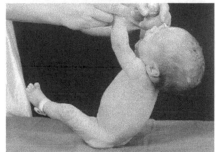

Fig. 6.19

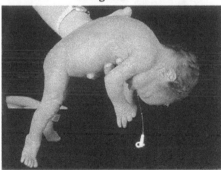

Fig. 6.16

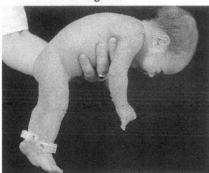

Fig. 6.20

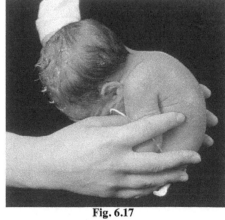

Fig. 6.17

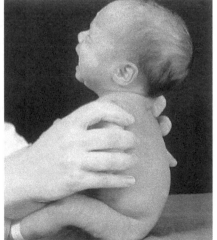

Fig. 6.21

113

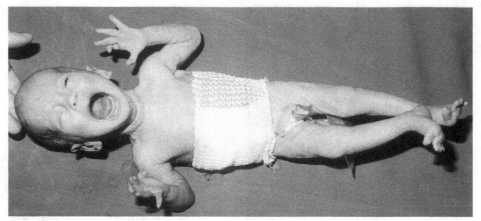

Fig. 6.22. Infant with subcortical leukomalacia at 40 weeks postmenstrual age, showing extreme irritability, marked arm flexion and leg extension, and persistently flexed left forefinger and extension of the big toes.

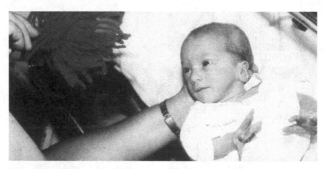

Fig. 6.23. Infant with mixed leukomalacia at 40 weeks postmenstrual age, showing an excellent tracking response.

Later, most infants with periventricular lesions become less irritable and develop signs of diplegia but maintain their vision (Fig. 6.24). Most infants with subcortical lesions remain irritable. In spite of their early good visual function, many subsequently develop severe visual impairment and, in many cases, infantile spasms and quadriplegia (Fig. 6.25). The evolution of abnormal signs in these infants illustrates the importance of repeated evaluations. If such infants are examined only around the time of discharge from the unit (often around 36 to 38 weeks postmenstrual age), they may well appear normal.

PERIVENTRICULAR LEUKOMALACIA IN COMPARISON WITH INTRAVENTRICULAR HAEMORRHAGE

During the stage of acute neonatal haemorrhage and leukomalacia, clinical signs are often fairly non-specific and are not likely to differentiate the two conditions. By the time the affected preterm infant reaches term age, however, the neurological examination shows a remarkable difference (Table 6.1).

Fig. 6.24.   Fig. 6.25.

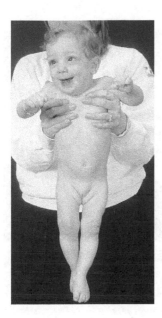

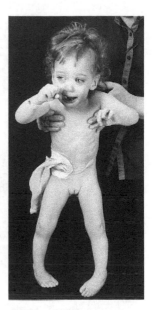

Figs. 6.24–6.25. Clinical outcome in an infant with cystic periventricular leukomalacia (PVL) (6.24) and one with subcortical leukomalacia (6.25). Whereas the child with PVL developed diplegia and became less irritable, the one with subcortical lesions developed quadriplegia and remained irritable.

TABLE 6.1
Clinical signs in preterm infants with multicystic periventricular leukomalacia (PVL) and large intraventricular haemorrhage (IVH) at 40 weeks postmenstrual age

	Multicystic PVL	*Large IVH*
Head and trunk control	N or ⇑	N or ⇓
Neck extension>flexion	++	±
Limb tone	⇑	N or ⇓
Asymmetry	–	++
Abnormal finger posture	+++	+
Motility	Abnormal	Variable
Tremors and startles	+++	+
Moro reflex	Mainly extension	Mainly abduction
Irritability	+++	+

N, normal; arrows indicate increase (⇑) or decrease (⇓) relative to normal findings.
±, +, ++, +++, relative strength of sign.

The difference can also be observed in Figures 6.26 to 6.33, which illustrate clinical neurological findings at term in twins born at 27 weeks gestation, one with IVH and the other with PVL, examined at term. While the infant with IVH showed flexion of the legs (Fig. 6.28), the one with PVL had an extended leg posture and a flexed arm posture (Fig. 6.29). IVH was associated with slightly decreased trunk tone on the ventral suspension test (Fig. 6.30) and PVL with increased trunk tone (Fig. 6.31). The infant with IVH showed no popliteal tightness (Fig. 6.32), while the twin with PVL showed smaller popliteal angles (Fig. 6.33). Fig. 6.34 shows the children at 9 months chronological age.

IVH   PVL

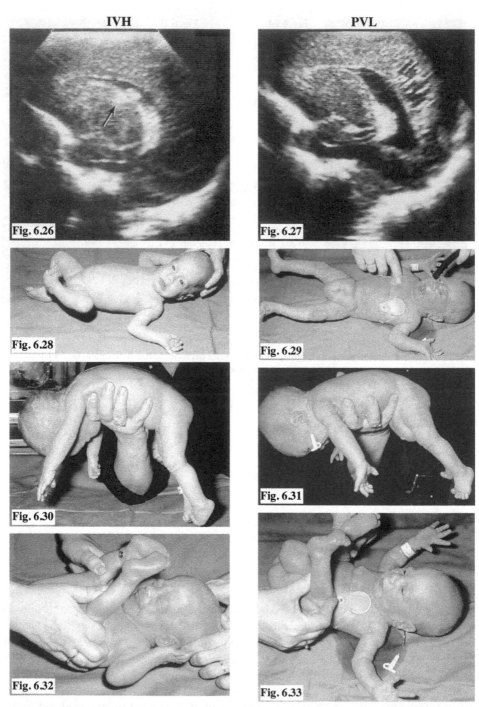

Figs. 6.26–6.33. Comparison of ultrasound findings and neurological findings in twins born at 27 weeks gestation, one with IVH (left) and one with PVL (right).

IVH   PVL

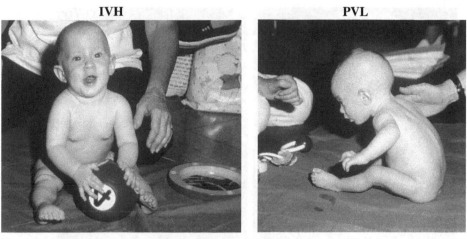

Fig. 6.34. Outcome in the twins shown in Figures 6.26–6.33 The one with IVH (*left*) is normal and the one with PVL (*right*) has cerebral palsy.

Cerebral infarction

Until recently, neonatal cerebral infarction was thought to be relatively uncommon, to be usually associated with perinatal complications, and to be associated with a very unfavourable outcome. The advent of routine brain imaging in the neonatal period has shown that cerebral infarction is a relatively common lesion, particularly in infants who do not have birth asphyxia but present with seizures in the first 48 hours of life (Mercuri et al. 1995, 1999). Most such infants show infarction of one or more branches of the middle cerebral artery, with the left hemisphere more frequently affected than the right.

The ultrasound abnormalities consist in localized densities involving the periventricular regions and/or the basal ganglia. They are best seen with a 5-MHz transducer and become more obvious on the scans performed at the end of the first week (Fig. 6.35).

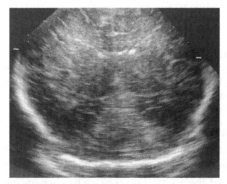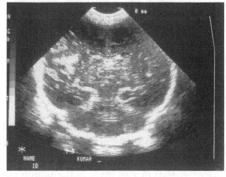

Fig. 6.35. Cranial ultrasound (coronal views) in a term infant at day 3 (*left*) and day 8 (*right*) after birth. Note that the increased echogenicity clearly seen at 5 MHz in the left parietal region on day 8 is much less visible on the initial ultrasound at 7.5 MHz on day 3.

117

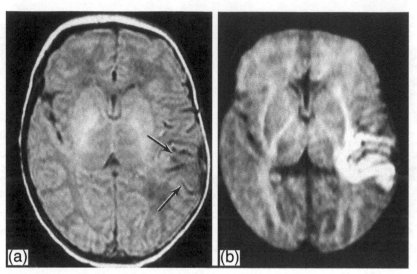

Fig. 6.36. MRI of same infant as in Fig. 6.35. A T₁-weighted sequence at 2 days of age (a) showed an area of low signal intensity in the left parietal lobe. The region of infarction is clearly demonstrated on the diffusion-weighted imaging as high signal intensity (b).

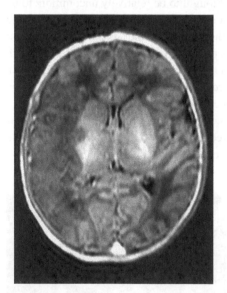

Fig. 6.37. MRI of male infant. A T₁-weighted sequence at 10 days of age showed an area of low signal intensity in the right parietal lobe involving the whole territory of the main branch of the middle cerebral artery.

The type and extent of the lesions can be seen better on MRI. Changes consist in loss of grey/white matter differentiation and abnormal signal in the area of the infarct, which can be localized in the territory of one of the cortical branches of the middle cerebral artery (Fig. 6.36a) or can involve the whole territory of the artery (Fig. 6.37). The changes can already be within a day after the insult by using diffusion-weighted imaging sequences (Fig. 6.36b) and can be clearly seen on conventional sequences at the end of the first week.

The initial neonatal examination can be quite variable, with findings ranging from normal to the presence of marked asymmetry in tone and movement. In most cases, the initial finding is of generalized hypotonia, but as most infants with cerebral infarction have convulsions and are being treated with anticonvulsant drugs, the significance of this finding is uncertain. Later, generally within a few weeks, some of these infants show some asymmetry of limb tone, which usually disappears by 2 to 3 months of age.

In our experience, clinical findings in newborn infants with neonatal infarction, whether normal or abnormal, offer little clue to the outcome: a normal examination in the neonatal period does not exclude the possibility of future hemiplegia, while early asymmetries (Fig. 6.40, overleaf) can be compatible with a completely normal outcome (Mercuri et al. 1999) (Figs. 6.41–6.45.

The EEG recorded in the first days after birth can provide better prognostic information. In our experience, all the children with a normal background activity, even if that is accompanied by epileptic discharges, have a normal outcome. In contrast, infants with a discontinuous background activity, either unilateral or bilateral, tend to have hemiplegia later on (Fig. 6.38).

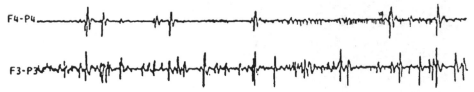

Fig. 6.38. Four-channel EEG of a newborn infant with focal infarction who later developed hemiplegia. Note that the background activity is asymmetrical.

Hypoxic–ischaemic encephalopathy

Perinatal hypoxic–ischaemic events are a major cause of morbidity and mortality in the term infant. The exact definition of which infants should be considered to have hypoxic–ischaemic encephalopathy (HIE) varies (Levene 1995). Our definition of an infant with HIE is one who shows neurological abnormalities in the first 48 hours of life, after evidence of fetal distress, i.e. meconium-stained liquor, and/or cardiotocographic abnormalities, and low Apgar scores (below 5 at 1 minute and below 8 at 5 minutes). The severity of HIE is usually classified according to the 3-point grading system suggested by Sarnat and Sarnat (1976) (Table 6.2, page 124).

Although the classification suggested by those authors is useful and very widely used, the difficulty has been the rather variable presentation and outcome in infants classified within a given stage, particularly stage-2 encephalopathy. There are various reasons for this. Clinical findings depend on when the examination is first performed, whether the infant has been treated with anticonvulsants, and the underlying pattern of brain lesions.

In recent years, using an integrated approach of clinical evaluation, imaging by ultrasound and magnetic resonance, and neurophysiological studies, we have been able to relate clinical imaging and neurophysiological findings. Although our cohort was relatively small, we were nevertheless able to define more specific patterns in relation to both lesions and outcome.

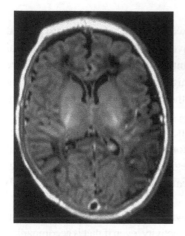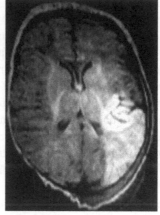

Fig. 6.39

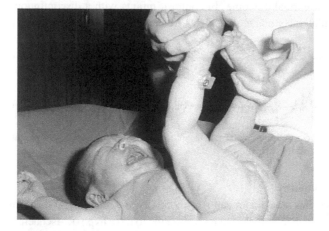

Fig. 6.40

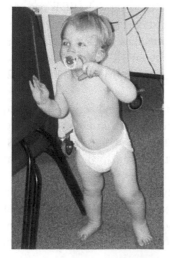

Fig. 6.41

Figs. 6.39–6.42. MRI scans (6.39) showing cerebral infarction in a male infant. The neurological examination performed on day 5 showed some asymmetry in arm traction, leg recoil, and leg traction (6.40 and *[facing page]* 6.42). At 15 months, the child did not show any sign of hemiplegia (6.41).

INFANT WITH INFARCTION – NORMAL OUTCOME

POSTURE Infant supine. Look mainly at position of legs but also note arms. *Score predominant posture.*	arms & legs extended or very slightly flexed	legs slightly flexed	legs well flexed but not adducted	legs well flexed & adducted near abdomen	abnormal posture: a) opisthotonus b) marked leg extension, strong arm flexion
ARM RECOIL Take both hands, quickly extend arms parallel to the body, Count to three. Release. Repeat 3 times.	arms do not flex	arms flex slowly, not always; not completely	arms flex slowly; more completely	arms flex quickly and completely	arms difficult to extend; snap back forcefully
ARM TRACTION Hold wrist and pull arm upwards. Note flexion at elbow and resistance while shoulder lifts off table. *Test each side separately.*	arms remain straight; no resistance felt	arms flex slightly or some resistance felt	arms flex well till shoulder lifts, then straighten	arms flex at approx 100° & maintained as shoulder lifts	flexion of arms <100°; maintained when body lifts up
LEG RECOIL Take *both* ankles in one hand, flex hips + knees. Quickly extend. Release. Repeat 3 times.	No flexion	incomplete or variable flexion	complete but slow flexion	complete fast flexion	legs difficult to extend; snap back forcefully
LEG TRACTION Grasp ankle and slowly pull leg upwards. Note flexion at knees and resistance as buttocks lift. *Test each side separately.*	legs straight - no resistance felt	legs flex slightly or some resistance felt	legs flex well till bottom lifts up	knee flexes remains flexed when bottom up	flexion stays when back+bottom up
POPLITEAL ANGLE Fix knee on abdomen, extend leg by gentle pressure with index finger behind the ankle. Note angle at knee. *Test each side separately.*	180°	≈150°	≈110°	≈90°	<90°
HEAD CONTROL (1) *(extensor tone)* Infant sitting upright. Encircle chest with both hands holding shoulders. Let head drop forward.	no attempt to raise head	infant tries: effort better felt than seen	raises head but drops forward or back	raises head: remains vertical; it may wobble	
HEAD CONTROL (2) *(flexor tone)* Infant sitting upright. Encircle chest with both hands holding shoulders. Let head drop backward.	no attempt to raise head	infant tries: effort better felt than seen	raises head but drops forward or back	raises head: remains vertical; it may wobble	head upright or extended; cannot be passively flexed
HEAD LAG Pull infant towards sitting posture by traction on both wrists & support head slightly. Also note arm flexion.	head drops & stays back	tries to lift head but it drops back	able to lift head slightly	lifts head in line with body	head in front of body
VENTRAL SUSPENSION Hold infant in ventral suspension. Observe back, flexion of limbs, and relation of head to trunk. If it looks different, DRAW.	back curved, head & limbs hang straight	back curved, head ↓, limbs slightly flexed	back slightly curved, limbs flexed	back straight, head in line, limbs flexed	back straight, head above body

Fig. 6.42

121

Fig. 6.43

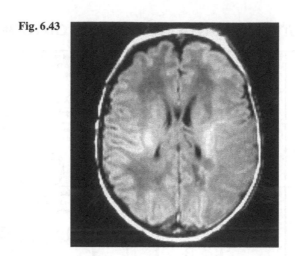

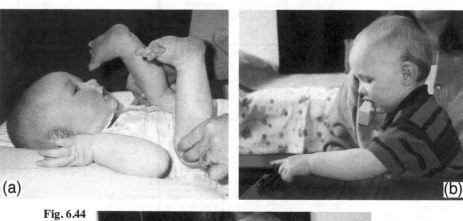

Fig. 6.44

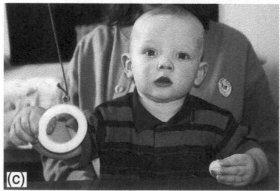

Figs. 6.43–6.45. MRI scan (6.43) in a male infant, showing an area of infarction similar to that detected in the infant in Figs. 6.39–6.41. The neurological examination on day 5 (6.44a; 6.45) showed some asymmetry in arm recoil, arm traction, leg traction, and popliteal angle. At 15 months, the child showed clear signs of right hemiplegia (6.44b,c).

INFANT WITH INFARCTION – HEMIPLEGIA

POSTURE Infant supine. Look mainly at position of legs but also note arms. *Score predominant posture.*	arms & legs extended or very slightly flexed	legs slightly flexed	legs well flexed but not adducted	legs well flexed & adducted near abdomen	abnormal posture: a) opisthotonus b) marked leg extension, strong arm flexion
ARM RECOIL Take both hands, quickly extend arms parallel to the body, Count to three. Release. Repeat 3 times.	arms do not flex	arms flex slowly, not always; not completely R	arms flex slowly; more completely L	arms flex quickly and completely	arms difficult to extend; snap back forcefully
ARM TRACTION Hold wrist and pull arm upwards. Note flexion at elbow and resistance while shoulder lifts off table. *Test each side separately.*	arms remain straight; no resistance felt R L	arms flex slightly or some resistance felt R	arms flex well till shoulder lifts, then straighten L	arms flex at approx 100° & maintained as shoulder lifts R L	flexion of arms <100°; maintained when body lifts up R L
LEG RECOIL Take *both* ankles in one hand, flex hips + knees. Quickly extend. Release. Repeat 3 times.	No flexion	incomplete or variable flexion	complete but slow flexion	complete fast flexion	legs difficult to extend; snap back forcefully
LEG TRACTION Grasp ankle and slowly pull leg upwards. Note flexion at knees and resistance as buttocks lift. *Test each side separately.*	legs straight - no resistance felt R L	legs flex slightly or some resistance felt R	legs flex well till bottom lifts up L	knee flexes remains flexed when bottom up R L	flexion stays when back+bottom up R L
POPLITEAL ANGLE Fix knee on abdomen, extend leg by gentle pressure with index finger behind the ankle. Note angle at knee. *Test each side separately.*	180° R L	≈150° R	≈110° L	≈90° R L	<90° R L
HEAD CONTROL (1) *(extensor tone)* Infant sitting upright. Encircle chest with both hands holding shoulders. Let head drop forward.	no attempt to raise head	infant tries: effort better felt than seen	raises head but drops forward or back	raises head: remains vertical; it may wobble	
HEAD CONTROL (2) *(flexor tone)* Infant sitting upright. Encircle chest with both hands holding shoulders. Let head drop backward.	no attempt to raise head	infant tries: effort better felt than seen	raises head but drops forward or back	raises head: remains vertical; it may wobble	head upright or extended; cannot be passively flexed
HEAD LAG Pull infant towards sitting posture by traction on both wrists & support head slightly. Also note arm flexion.	head drops & stays back	tries to lift head but it drops back	able to lift head slightly	lifts head in line with body	head in front of body
VENTRAL SUSPENSION Hold infant in ventral suspension. Observe back, flexion of limbs, and relation of head to trunk. If it looks different, DRAW.	back curved, head & limbs hang straight	back curved, head ↓, limbs slightly flexed	back slightly curved, limbs flexed	back straight, head in line, limbs flexed	back straight, head above body

Fig. 6.45

TABLE 6.2
Grading of neonatal hypoxic–ischaemic encephalopathy (HIE)[a]

	Mild (HIE I)	Moderate (HIE 2)	Severe (HIE 3)
Level of consciousness	Hyperalert	Lethargic	Stuporous
Neuromuscular control			
Muscle tone	Normal	Mild hypotonia	Flaccid
Posture	Mild distal flexion	Strong distal flexion	Intermittent decerebration
Stretch reflexes	Overactive	Overactive	Decreased or absent
Segmental myoclonus	Present	Present	Absent
Complex reflexes			
Sucking	Weak	Weak or absent	Absent
Moro	Strong, low threshold	Weak, high threshold	Absent
Oculovestibular	Normal	Overactive	Weak or absent
Tonic neck	Slight	Strong	Absent
Autonomic functions	Generalized sympathetic	Generalized parasympathetic	Both systems depressed
Pupils	Mydriasis	Miosis	Variable
Heart rate	Tachycardia	Bradycardia	Variable
Bronchial secretions	Sparse	Profuse	Variable
Gastrointestinal motility	Normal or decreased	Increased, diarrhoea	Variable
Seizures	None	Common	Uncommon (excluding decerebration)

[a] Classification of Sarnat and Sarnat (1976).

In the next section, we describe some of our findings in relation to the various stages of encephalopathy

HIE 1

Infants in this category often present with a history of some adverse antenatal or perinatal event. Their tone pattern may be near normal initially, but most have somewhat diminished axial tone, with extensor tone being better than flexor tone. They often show some thumb adduction or mild fisting and may be jittery. Although they have a good sucking reflex, they may have feeding difficulties. They are visually and auditorily hyperalert and often irritable. They normalize rapidly but may still have relatively poor head control, even at 3 to 6 weeks.

Cranial ultrasound findings in these infants may be completely normal or may show some mild periventricular densities or small intraventricular haemorrhages. The initial MRI may be normal or show mild brain swelling consistent with oedema. In addition, signal changes in the white matter may be found, but the signal intensity in the internal capsule is normal (Rutherford et al. 1998).

The early EEG shows a normal background activity; some sharp waves may be present. For these infants the outcome at 2 to 4 years is usually completely normal.

HIE 2

HIE 2 in our cohort encompassed a wide variety of clinical patterns. At one end of the scale are infants with a history and initial findings very similar to those for infants with stage-1 encephalopathy but who have also had a convulsive episode. In the infants with convulsions, treatment with anticonvulsants often makes them unresponsive and hypotonic (Fig. 6.46).

HIE 2 – MILD OEDEMA – DAY 3

POSTURE Infant supine. Look mainly at position of legs but also note arms. *Score predominant posture.*	arms & legs extended or very slightly flexed	legs slightly flexed	legs well flexed but not adducted	legs well flexed & adducted near abdomen	abnormal posture: a) opisthotonus b) marked leg extension, strong arm flexion
ARM RECOIL Take both hands, quickly extend arms parallel to the body, Count to three. Release. Repeat 3 times.	arms do not flex	arms flex slowly, not always; not completely	arms flex slowly; more completely	arms flex quickly and completely	arms difficult to extend; snap back forcefully
ARM TRACTION Hold wrist and pull arm upwards. Note flexion at elbow and resistance while shoulder lifts off table. *Test each side separately.*	arms remain straight; no resistance felt	arms flex slightly or some resistance felt	arms flex well till shoulder lifts, then straighten	arms flex at approx 100° & maintained as shoulder lifts	flexion of arms <100°; maintained when body lifts up
LEG RECOIL Take *both* ankles in one hand, flex hips + knees. Quickly extend. Release. Repeat 3 times.	No flexion	incomplete or variable flexion	complete but slow flexion	complete fast flexion	legs difficult to extend; snap back forcefully
LEG TRACTION Grasp ankle and slowly pull leg upwards. Note flexion at knees and resistance as buttocks lift. *Test each side separately.*	legs straight - no resistance felt	legs flex slightly or some resistance felt	legs flex well till bottom lifts up	knee flexes remains flexed when bottom up	flexion stays when back+bottom up
POPLITEAL ANGLE Fix knee on abdomen, extend leg by gentle pressure with index finger behind the ankle. Note angle at knee. *Test each side separately.*	180°	≈150°	≈110°	≈90°	<90°
HEAD CONTROL (1) *(extensor tone)* Infant sitting upright. Encircle chest with both hands holding shoulders. Let head drop forward.	no attempt to raise head	infant tries: effort better felt than seen	raises head but drops forward or back	raises head: remains vertical; it may wobble	
HEAD CONTROL (2) *(flexor tone)* Infant sitting upright. Encircle chest with both hands holding shoulders. Let head drop backward.	no attempt to raise head	infant tries: effort better felt than seen	raises head but drops forward or back	raises head: remains vertical; it may wobble	head upright or extended; cannot be passively flexed
HEAD LAG Pull infant towards sitting posture by traction on both wrists & support head slightly. Also note arm flexion.	head drops & stays back	tries to lift head but it drops back	able to lift head slightly	lifts head in line with body	head in front of body
VENTRAL SUSPENSION Hold infant in ventral suspension. Observe back, flexion of limbs, and relation of head to trunk. If it looks different, DRAW.	back curved, head & limbs hang straight	back curved, head ↓, limbs slightly flexed	back slightly curved, limbs flexed	back straight, head in line, limbs flexed	back straight, head above body

Fig. 6.46. Neurological examination performed on day 3 in a term infant with HIE 2 showing mild oedema on the initial MRI. Note that the tone on the items assessing leg recoil and leg traction was slightly reduced for her gestational age. This infant appeared normal in alertness, sucking reflex, and other reflexes.

125

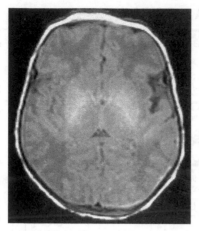

Fig. 6.47. MRI scan (inversion recovery sequence) showing mild, generalized brain oedema on day 2 in an infant with HIE 2.

Some infants also have other associated medical problems such as meconium aspiration with pulmonary hypertension, cardiac problems, or renal problems. They may show poor tone and responsiveness due to non-neurological causes, and the whole clinical picture can become very confusing. All these infants are slower to recover than those with HIE 1 and may remain hypotonic even longer than 3 to 6 weeks of age.

The ultrasound and MRI findings (Fig. 6.47) are similar to those for infants with HIE 1. The EEG may show epileptiform discharges but a normal background. The outcome is similar to that for infants with HIE 1.

At the other end of the scale are two other categories. The first comprises infants who present with more severe antenatal problems, such as reduced fetal growth associated with reduced fetal movement, and who have superadded perinatal problems such as fetal distress. The second category comprises infants who had a normal antenatal course but sustained a severe, sudden, acute event around the time of delivery, such as placental abruption, a ruptured uterus, cord prolapse, or a prolonged, difficult delivery with severe fetal distress.

On the whole, the infants with predominantly antenatal problems are at first markedly hypotonic, have adducted thumbs or fisting, and are not jittery. They can suck and swallow, but they suck slowly and therefore feed slowly. Their auditory response is usually good but their visual alertness is poor and they are not particularly irritable (Fig. 6.48). They have convulsions and often are treated with quite powerful anticonvulsants, so that it is always difficult to judge how much of their depressed state is attributable to the treatment and how much to the encephalopathy. Usually after the end of the second week these infants show good recovery. Their tone improves: head control is still poor, but the limbs have good flexor tone. Adduction of the thumbs tends to persist, and spontaneously upgoing toes may also be observed (Fig. 6.49). At this stage, the infants may become jittery and they may be quite irritable. Their sucking and feeding is much improved and therefore they are usually able to feed entirely from bottle or breast. They are more alert than before, with quite good visual orientation. Their condition improves rapidly after this and by 4 to 6 weeks may differ very little from that of the infants with milder initial signs (Fig. 6.50) (Mercuri et al. 1999b).

	arms & legs extended or very slightly flexed	legs slightly flexed	legs well flexed but not adducted	legs well flexed & adducted near abdomen	abnormal posture: a) opisthotonus b) marked leg extension, strong arm flexion
POSTURE Infant supine. Look mainly at position of legs but also note arms. *Score predominant posture.*					
ARM RECOIL Take both hands, quickly extend arms parallel to the body, Count to three. Release. Repeat 3 times.	arms do not flex	arms flex slowly, not always; not completely	arms flex slowly; more completely	arms flex quickly and completely	arms difficult to extend; snap back forcefully
ARM TRACTION Hold wrist and pull arm upwards. Note flexion at elbow and resistance while shoulder lifts off table. *Test each side separately.*	arms remain straight; no resistance felt	arms flex slightly or some resistance felt	arms flex well till shoulder lifts, then straighten	arms flex at approx 100° & maintained as shoulder lifts	flexion of arms <100°; maintained when body lifts up
LEG RECOIL Take *both* ankles in one hand, flex hips + knees. Quickly extend. Release. Repeat 3 times.	No flexion	incomplete or variable flexion	complete but slow flexion	complete fast flexion	legs difficult to extend; snap back forcefully
LEG TRACTION Grasp ankle and slowly pull leg upwards. Note flexion at knees and resistance as buttocks lift. *Test each side separately.*	legs straight - no resistance felt	legs flex slightly or some resistance felt	legs flex well till bottom lifts up	knee flexes remains flexed when bottom up	flexion stays when back+bottom up
POPLITEAL ANGLE Fix knee on abdomen, extend leg by gentle pressure with index finger behind the ankle. Note angle at knee. *Test each side separately.*	180°	≈150°	≈110°	≈90°	<90°
HEAD CONTROL (1) *(extensor tone)* Infant sitting upright. Encircle chest with both hands holding shoulders. Let head drop forward.	no attempt to raise head	infant tries: effort better felt than seen	raises head but drops forward or back	raises head: remains vertical; it may wobble	
HEAD CONTROL (2) *(flexor tone)* Infant sitting upright. Encircle chest with both hands holding shoulders. Let head drop backward.	no attempt to raise head	infant tries: effort better felt than seen	raises head but drops forward or back	raises head: remains vertical; it may wobble	head upright or extended; cannot be passively flexed
HEAD LAG Pull infant towards sitting posture by traction on both wrists & support head slightly. Also note arm flexion.	head drops & stays back	tries to lift head but it drops back	able to lift head slightly	lifts head in line with body	head in front of body
VENTRAL SUSPENSION Hold infant in ventral suspension. Observe back, flexion of limbs, and relation of head to trunk. If it looks different, DRAW.	back curved, head & limbs hang straight	back curved, head ↓, limbs slightly flexed	back slightly curved, limbs flexed	back straight, head in line, limbs flexed	back straight, head above body

Fig. 6.48 *(continues overleaf)*

TREMOR		no tremor, or tremor only when crying or only after Moro reflex	tremor occasionally when awake	frequent tremors when awake	continuous tremors
VISUAL ORIENTATION Wrap infant, wake up with rattle if needed or rock gently. Note if baby can see and follow red ball (B) or target (T). B T	does not follow or focus on stimuli B T	stills, focuses, follows briefly to the side but loses stimuli B T	follows horizontally and vertically; no head turn B T	follows horizontally and vertically; turns head B T	follows in a circle B T
IRRITABILITY In response to stimuli.	quiet all the time, not irritable to any stimuli	awakes, cries sometimes when handled	cries often when handled	cries always when handled	cries even when not handled

Fig. 6.48 (*above and overleaf*). Neurological examination on day 6 in a term infant with HIE 2 who suffered predominantly antenatal problems and in whom MRI showed diffuse white matter changes and relatively spared basal ganglia. He was generally hypotonic but had no tremors and had relatively preserved visual orientation. He also showed continuous adduction of the thumbs and a poor sucking reflex. The Moro and placing reflexes were present but incomplete. The infant's movements were sluggish and uncoordinated. See also Fig. 6.50.

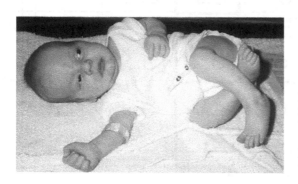

Fig. 6.49. Term infant with HIE 2 who had mainly antenatal problems, examined after the end of the second week. His posture shows relatively preserved flexor tone, upgoing big toes, and an adducted thumb. (Cf. Fig. 6.51.)

HIE 2 – 'ANTENATAL' PROBLEMS – 5 WEEKS

TREMOR		no tremor, or tremor only when crying or only after Moro reflex	tremor occasionally when awake	frequent tremors when awake	continuous tremors
VISUAL ORIENTATION Wrap infant, wake up with rattle if needed or rock gently. Note if baby can see and follow red ball (B) or target (T). B T	does not follow or focus on stimuli B T	stills, focuses, follows briefly to the side but loses stimuli B T	follows horizontally and vertically; no head turn B T	follows horizontally and vertically; turns head B T	follows in a circle B T
IRRITABILITY In response to stimuli.	quiet all the time, not irritable to any stimuli	awakes, cries sometimes when handled	cries often when handled	cries always when handled	cries even when not handled

Fig. 6.50 (*above and facing page*). Neurological findings for same infant as in Fig. 6.48. At 5 weeks, the infant's tone had improved. He still showed intermittent adduction of the thumbs. Visual orientation and the sucking, placing, and Moro reflexes were all normal. He had some smooth alternating movements, but frequent stretching and jerky movements were also present.

POSTURE Infant supine. Look mainly at position of legs but also note arms. *Score predominant posture.*	arms & legs extended or very slightly flexed	legs slightly flexed	legs well flexed but not adducted	legs well flexed & adducted near abdomen	abnormal posture: a) opisthotonus b) marked leg extension, strong arm flexion		
ARM RECOIL Take both hands, quickly extend arms parallel to the body, Count to three. Release. Repeat 3 times.	arms do not flex	arms flex slowly, not always; not completely	arms flex slowly; more completely	arms flex quickly and completely	arms difficult to extend; snap back forcefully		
ARM TRACTION Hold wrist and pull arm upwards. Note flexion at elbow and resistance while shoulder lifts off table. *Test each side separately.*	arms remain straight; no resistance felt	arms flex slightly or some resistance felt	arms flex well till shoulder lifts, then straighten	arms flex at approx 100° & maintained as shoulder lifts	flexion of arms <100°; maintained when body lifts up		
LEG RECOIL Take *both* ankles in one hand, flex hips + knees. Quickly extend. Release. Repeat 3 times.	No flexion	incomplete or variable flexion	complete but slow flexion	complete fast flexion	legs difficult to extend; snap back forcefully		
LEG TRACTION Grasp ankle and slowly pull leg upwards. Note flexion at knees and resistance as buttocks lift. *Test each side separately.*	legs straight - no resistance felt	legs flex slightly or some resistance felt	legs flex well till bottom lifts up	knee flexes remains flexed when bottom up	flexion stays when back+bottom up		
POPLITEAL ANGLE Fix knee on abdomen, extend leg by gentle pressure with index finger behind the ankle. Note angle at knee. *Test each side separately.*	100°	≈150°	≈110°	≈90°	<90°		
HEAD CONTROL (1) *(extensor tone)* Infant sitting upright. Encircle chest with both hands holding shoulders. Let head drop forward.	no attempt to raise head	infant tries: effort better felt than seen	raises head but drops forward or back	raises head: remains vertical; it may wobble			
HEAD CONTROL (2) *(flexor tone)* Infant sitting upright. Encircle chest with both hands holding shoulders. Let head drop backward.	no attempt to raise head	infant tries: effort better felt than seen	raises head but drops forward or back	raises head: remains vertical; it may wobble	head upright or extended; cannot be passively flexed		
HEAD LAG Pull infant towards sitting posture by traction on both wrists & support head slightly. Also note arm flexion.	head drops & stays back	tries to lift head but it drops back	able to lift head slightly	lifts head in line with body	head in front of body		
VENTRAL SUSPENSION Hold infant in ventral suspension. Observe back, flexion of limbs, and relation of head to trunk. If it looks different, DRAW.	back curved, head & limbs hang straight	back curved, head ↓, limbs slightly flexed	back slightly curved, limbs flexed	back straight, head in line, limbs flexed	back straight, head above body		

Fig. 6.50, *continued*

129

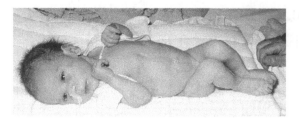

Fig. 6.51. Term infant with HIE 2 who had experienced severe, acute perinatal events, examined at the end of the second week. Note the posture with partial extension of the legs and marked flexion in the arms, and the toes curling under the feet. (Cf. Fig. 6.49).

The other category of infants – the ones who had no antenatal problems but who suffered a severe, acute perinatal asphyxial event – also present initially with marked hypotonia and fisting, but the toes, instead of being extended, tend to curl under (Fig.6.51). These infants cannot suck and often have difficulty in swallowing. They have very poor alertness, with poor auditory orientation and an inability to fixate and focus visually. At this stage they are not irritable and cry only rarely. During the next 2 weeks a different clinical picture emerges. Although the hypotonia may persist, they often lie in an extended posture, with extension of the legs and marked flexion of the arms. Increased extensor tone in the neck develops and becomes more and more marked. In addition, dystonic posturing may often be noted, with frequent tremors and jerky movement. Cycling movement and other abnormal movements resembling convulsions are frequent, but these are often not associated with epileptic discharges. Movements in general are stereotyped and cramped. The infants cannot suck and they swallow only poorly. Frequent abnormal eye movements can be observed. Although the infants may appear alert, they cannot fixate and follow visually (Fig. 6.52). When they are seen after 5 weeks, many of the abnormal tone patterns and movements are even more prominent (Fig. 6.53). The infants remain unable to feed from either breast or bottle. They still cannot fixate or focus visually. They often are very irritable. Convulsions are frequently present and are often resistant to treatment.

The initial cranial ultrasound (day 1 to 2) is likely to show loss of definition both in the children with predominantly antenatal problems and in the ones with acute insults. However, on later ultrasound examination (day 4 to 5), the infants with predominantly antenatal problems show marked periventricular densities, whereas in the ones who have sustained acute insults, echogenic areas in the basal ganglia are observed. Some periventricular echogenic features may also be present, but these are not prominent.

The initial marked brain swelling seen on MRI scans is also similar in the two groups. When the oedema subsides, however, the patterns of lesions are quite different. Infants with antenatal problems are likely to show extensive signal changes in the white matter, with associated cortical highlighting. Some basal ganglia changes may be noted, but these are often unilateral or relatively transient. The signal in the internal capsule is abnormal but may normalize relatively rapidly (6.54a,b,c). In infants with more acute insults, in contrast, the most striking changes are in the basal ganglia and thalami, with complete absence of signal from myelin in the internal capsule (Fig. 6.55a,b,c). The white matter is often streaky. Some cortical highlighting may be present, but this tends to be less marked than that seen in the group with antenatal onset.

HIE 2 – 'PERINATAL' PROBLEMS – DAY 7

POSTURE Infant supine. Look mainly at position of legs but also note arms. *Score predominant posture.*	arms & legs extended or very slightly flexed	legs slightly flexed	legs well flexed but not adducted	legs well flexed & adducted near abdomen	abnormal posture: a) opisthotonus b) marked leg extension, strong arm flexion
ARM RECOIL Take both hands, quickly extend arms parallel to the body, Count to three. Release. Repeat 3 times.	arms do not flex	arms flex slowly, not always; not completely	arms flex slowly; more completely	arms flex quickly and completely	arms difficult to extend; snap back forcefully
ARM TRACTION Hold wrist and pull arm upwards. Note flexion at elbow and resistance while shoulder lifts off table. *Test each side separately.*	arms remain straight; no resistance felt	arms flex slightly or some resistance felt	arms flex well till shoulder lifts, then straighten	arms flex at approx 100° & maintained as shoulder lifts	flexion of arms <100°; maintained when body lifts up
LEG RECOIL Take *both* ankles in one hand, flex hips + knees. Quickly extend. Release. Repeat 3 times.	No flexion	incomplete or variable flexion	complete but slow flexion	complete fast flexion	legs difficult to extend; snap back forcefully
LEG TRACTION Grasp ankle and slowly pull leg upwards. Note flexion at knees and resistance as buttocks lift. *Test each side separately.*	legs straight - no resistance felt	legs flex slightly or some resistance felt	legs flex well till bottom lifts up	knee flexes remains flexed when bottom up	flexion stays when back+bottom up
POPLITEAL ANGLE Fix knee on abdomen, extend leg by gentle pressure with index finger behind the ankle. Note angle at knee. *Test each side separately.*	180°	≈150°	≈110°	≈90°	<90°
HEAD CONTROL (1) *(extensor tone)* Infant sitting upright. Encircle chest with both hands holding shoulders. Let head drop forward.	no attempt to raise head	infant tries: effort better felt than seen	raises head but drops forward or back	raises head: remains vertical; it may wobble	
HEAD CONTROL (2) *(flexor tone)* Infant sitting upright. Encircle chest with both hands holding shoulders. Let head drop backward.	no attempt to raise head	infant tries: effort better felt than seen	raises head but drops forward or back	raises head: remains vertical; it may wobble	head upright or extended; cannot be passively flexed
HEAD LAG Pull infant towards sitting posture by traction on both wrists & support head slightly. Also note arm flexion.	head drops & stays back	tries to lift head but it drops back	able to lift head slightly	lifts head in line with body	head in front of body
VENTRAL SUSPENSION Hold infant in ventral suspension. Observe back, flexion of limbs, and relation of head to trunk. If it looks different, DRAW.	back curved, head & limbs hang straight	back curved, head ↓, limbs slightly flexed	back slightly curved, limbs flexed	back straight, head in line, limbs flexed	back straight, head above body

Fig. 6.52(*continues overleaf*)

131

HIE 2 – 'PERINATAL' PROBLEMS – DAY 7 *(cont'd.)*

TREMOR		no tremor, or tremor only when crying or only after Moro reflex	tremor occasionally when awake	frequent tremors when awake	continuous tremors
VISUAL ORIENTATION Wrap infant, wake up with rattle if needed or rock gently. Note if baby can see and follow red ball (B) or target (T).	does not follow or focus on stimuli B T	stills, focuses, follows briefly to the side but loses stimuli B T	follows horizontally and vertically; no head turn B T	follows horizontally and vertically; turns head B T	follows in a circle B T
IRRITABILITY In response to stimuli.	quiet all the time, not irritable to any stimuli	awakes, cries sometimes when handled	cries often when handled	cries always when handled	cries even when not handled

Fig. 6.52 *(above and facing page).* Neurological examination on day 7 in a female term infant with HIE 2 who had sustained severe, acute perinatal insults. She was generally hypotonic, had continuous unilateral adduction of a thumb, and had a few tremors. Visual orientation was absent. The child was unresponsive and had a poor sucking reflex and no Moro or placing reflex. Her movements were sluggish and uncoordinated, with some repetitive cycling movements and mouthing.

The outcome in infants with HIE 2 varies greatly, ranging from normal to severe cerebral palsy. The initial neurological examination gives only limited information, as it can be partly affected by medication or by non-neurological causes. However, repeated neurological examination in the neonatal period can provide important prognostic information. In our cohort, the speed of recovery was a reliable prognostic indicator. All the infants whose neurological examination normalized within 2 weeks had a normal outcome, whereas the ones who were consistently abnormal after 3 to 4 weeks all had an abnormal outcome.

The combined use of MRI allows more specific information on the types of sequelae these children are likely to develop. Children whose MRI scans are normal by the end of the first week are likely to have a normal outcome.

HIE 2 – 'PERINATAL' PROBLEMS – 5 WEEKS

TREMOR		no tremor, or tremor only when crying or only after Moro reflex	tremor occasionally when awake	frequent tremors when awake	continuous tremors
VISUAL ORIENTATION Wrap infant, wake up with rattle if needed or rock gently. Note if baby can see and follow red ball (B) or target (T).	does not follow or focus on stimuli B T	stills, focuses, follows briefly to the side but loses stimuli B T	follows horizontally and vertically; no head turn B T	follows horizontally and vertically; turns head B T	follows in a circle B T
IRRITABILITY In response to stimuli.	quiet all the time, not irritable to any stimuli	awakes, cries sometimes when handled	cries often when handled	cries always when handled	cries even when not handled

Fig. 6.53 *(facing page and above).* Neurological examination at 5 weeks of same infant as in Fig. 6.52. At this age the infant developed increased extensor tone, observable in the posture, in the difference between head flexion and extension, and in her poor response on the head lag test compared with that on ventral suspension. At this age, she still had continuous hand fisting. Her sucking, Moro, and placing reflexes were all poor. Her visual orientation was also still very poor and she was very irritable. Her motility was excessive, with uncoordinated movements.

POSTURE Infant supine. Look mainly at position of legs but also note arms. *Score predominant posture.*	arms & legs extended or very slightly flexed	legs slightly flexed	legs well flexed but not adducted	legs well flexed & adducted near abdomen	abnormal posture: a) opisthotonus b) marked leg extension, strong arm flexion		
ARM RECOIL Take both hands, quickly extend arms parallel to the body, Count to three. Release. Repeat 3 times.	arms do not flex	arms flex slowly, not always; not completely	arms flex slowly; more completely	arms flex quickly and completely	arms difficult to extend; snap back forcefully		
ARM TRACTION Hold wrist and pull arm upwards. Note flexion at elbow and resistance while shoulder lifts off table. *Test each side separately.*	arms remain straight; no resistance felt	arms flex slightly or some resistance felt	arms flex well till shoulder lifts, then straighten	arms flex at approx 100° & maintained as shoulder lifts	flexion of arms <100°; maintained when body lifts up		
LEG RECOIL Take *both* ankles in one hand, flex hips + knees. Quickly extend. Release. Repeat 3 times.	No flexion	incomplete or variable flexion	complete but slow flexion	complete fast flexion	legs difficult to extend; snap back forcefully		
LEG TRACTION Grasp ankle and slowly pull leg upwards. Note flexion at knees and resistance as buttocks lift. *Test each side separately.*	legs straight - no resistance felt	legs flex slightly or some resistance felt	legs flex well till bottom lifts up	knee flexes remains flexed when bottom up	flexion stays when back+bottom up		
POPLITEAL ANGLE Fix knee on abdomen, extend leg by gentle pressure with index finger behind the ankle. Note angle at knee. *Test each side separately.*	180°	~ 150°	≈110°	≈90°	<90°		
HEAD CONTROL (1) *(extensor tone)* Infant sitting upright. Encircle chest with both hands holding shoulders. Let head drop forward.	no attempt to raise head	infant tries: effort better felt than seen	raises head but drops forward or back	raises head: remains vertical; it may wobble			
HEAD CONTROL (2) *(flexor tone)* Infant sitting upright. Encircle chest with both hands holding shoulders. Let head drop backward.	no attempt to raise head	infant tries: effort better felt than seen	raises head but drops forward or back	raises head: remains vertical; It may wobble	head upright or extended; cannot be passively flexed		
HEAD LAG Pull infant towards sitting posture by traction on both wrists & support head slightly. Also note arm flexion.	head drops & stays back	tries to lift head but it drops back	able to lift head slightly	lifts head in line with body	head in front of body		
VENTRAL SUSPENSION Hold infant in ventral suspension. Observe back, flexion of limbs, and relation of head to trunk. If it looks different, DRAW.	back curved, head & limbs hang straight	back curved, head ↓, limbs slightly flexed	back slightly curved, limbs flexed	back straight, head in line, limbs flexed	back straight, head above body		

133

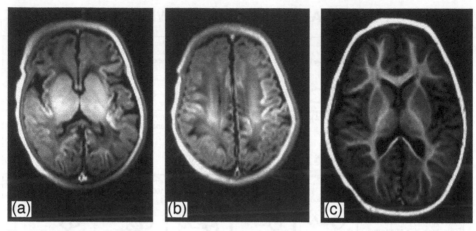

Fig. 6.54. MRI scans (inversion recovery) in a female term infant with HIE 2 who had had mainly antenatal problems. On day 20, there was some localized excessive increased signal intensity in the right lentiform nucleus (a) and increased highlighting of the cortex (a, b), most prominent in the insula and around the central fissure. This is most prominent at the depth of the sulci. There is adjacent decreased signal intensity in the subcortical white matter. At 18 months (c), there is delayed myelination, decreased volume of the white matter, and thin corpus callosum posteriorly. The basal ganglia show no focal abnormalities.

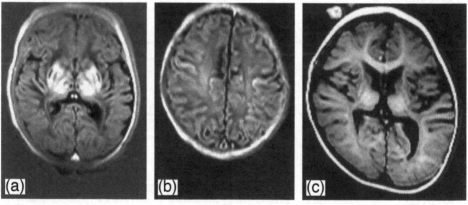

Fig. 6.55. MRI scans (inversion recovery) in a female term infant with HIE 2 who had experienced severe, acute perinatal insults. At 23 days, she had a marked abnormal high signal throughout the basal ganglia and thalami (a) and only mild highlighting of the cortex (a, b), with low signal in the adjacent white matter. At 15 months (c), she showed marked atrophy of the basal ganglia, thalami, and white matter. The ventricles are mildly dilated, with an irregular outline.

Children with predominantly antenatal problems and diffuse white matter changes usually develop microcephaly, cerebral palsy, and mild to moderate global delay (Fig. 6.56). The severity of the outcome seems to depend largely on the extent of the basal ganglia

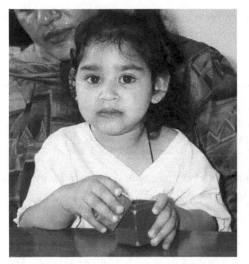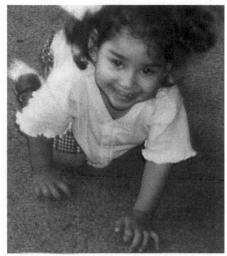

Fig. 6.56. Child with diffuse white matter changes but no significant basal ganglia involvement at 2 years of age. (See MRI, Fig. 6.54.)

Fig. 6.57. Child with diffuse basal ganglia lesions showing dystonic cerebral palsy and severe global delay. (See MRI, Fig. 6.55.)

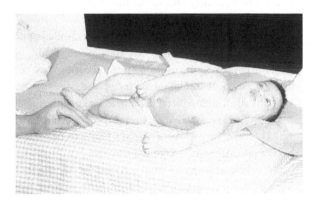

involvement. When the basal ganglia are spared or relatively little involved, the children will eventually be able to walk and their cognitive delay is generally milder.

The severity of the outcome for children with more acute perinatal insults also seems to depend on the extent of the basal ganglia involvement. The infants with more severe and diffuse basal ganglia lesions develop microcephaly, dystonic cerebral palsy, and severe global delay, often showing no discernible development (Fig. 6.57). In contrast, infants with more discrete basal ganglia lesions generally develop athetoid cerebral palsy but have a normal head circumference and normal cognitive development.

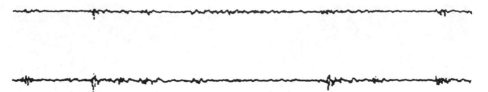

Fig. 6.58. Four-channel EEG in a newborn term infant with HIE who had sustained severe, acute perinatal insults and who had severe basal ganglia lesions. Note that the background activity is of extremely low amplitude.

The EEG shows an abnormal background with various degrees of discontinuity, more marked in the infants with acute insults (Fig. 6.58).

HIE 3

Infants with HIE 3 usually present with a catastrophic event around the time of delivery or soon after. Such infants may or may not have a history of an earlier antenatal event. They are initially comatose, flaccid, and unresponsive, breathe irregularly, and often require ventilation. If they regain consciousness and survive, their clinical signs during the recovery phase are basically similar to those of the infants with grade 2 encephalopathy with predominantly basal ganglia lesions.

On the initial ultrasound, a "snowstorm-like" appearance is often noted, and structures cannot be identified. When this appearance clears, widespread echogenic features in the thalami, basal ganglia, white matter, and cortex may be noted. The initial MRI shows marked brain oedema. If the infant survives, widespread changes can be seen in the cortical and subcortical structures. The thalami, basal ganglia, and cortex are always heavily involved.

The EEG is usually of extremely low amplitude.

Those infants who survive are likely to become quadriplegic, with dystonic cerebral palsy and extremely severe global delay.

As the foregoing section makes clear, the three stages of HIE defined by Sarnat and Sarnat (1976) constitute a spectrum, with an overlap in pattern of lesions and in outcome.

7
ADAPTATION OF THE NEUROLOGICAL PROFORMA

One advantage of our methodology is that it can easily be adapted or modified to meet the needs of specific circumstances. To illustrate this point, we discuss in this chapter some of the modifications we have made to adapt the proforma for specific circumstances and which are presently under pilot study. The principal adaptations are as (i) a screening tool for the routine examination of newborn infants in the maternity ward or at their first postnatal follow-up and (ii) an examination for use in developing countries. We also illustrate how we used the principles of the methodology of the neonatal examination to design a follow-up examination for infants, to enable relatively inexperienced staff to achieve objective recording of basic neurological signs and developmental milestones in a busy routine-follow-up clinic.

A neurological screening test for general use in term infants
Ideally, every newborn infant should have a comprehensive neurological examination; in practice, this certainly does not happen. In hospitals with many deliveries and frequent staff shortages, term infants usually receive a general medical examination, which includes only a few neurological items such as a general statement on tone, alertness, and the Moro reflex. The items are customarily ticked to denote normality, and only findings that the examiner considers grossly abnormal are listed. The problem arises if the same infant later presents with some abnormal neurological sign, such as a convulsion. It may be practically impossible to gauge from the forms, even if they are filled in, whether the infant was completely normal at the time of the first examination or whether even at that time some deviant signs were present. From a practical point of view, both in relation to aetiology and to prognosis, these early findings could be very important.

To make it possible to record the neurological status of each newborn infant more fully and more accurately, we have developed a shorter, simplified version of the proforma, which can be completed even if only very limited time is available for each examination. This should ensure more objective recordings of the routine clinical examination of the new-born infant, even by less-experienced or overextended staff, and should also help to raise some alarm bells and flag the potentially abnormal infant. This form is illustrated in Figure 7.1.

An adaptation of this form is now also being piloted in South Africa as part of a screening program for 6-week-old infants.

Adaptation of the neurological proforma for developing countries
There are many reasons why one would wish to have a neonatal neurological examination that can be widely used in developing countries. Although birth asphyxia is much more

Neurological screening proforma for term neonates

Name   DOB   Age at exam

Fontanelle   Head circumference

Limb tone

	ABNORMAL	OPTIMAL	ABNORMAL/DEVIANT	COMMENTS
POSTURE Baby lying supine. Look mainly at position of legs but also note arms. *You may change the drawing.*	arms & legs extended	leg well flexed but not adducted	opisthotonous or arm very flexed, leg very extended	
ARM TRACTION Hold wrist and pull upwards. Note flexion at arm and resistance while shoulder lifts off table.	arms remain straight - no resistance	arms flex and remain flexed as shoulders lift	arms remain flexed when body lifts up	
LEG TRACTION Hold ankle, pull leg upwards. Look at flexion & resistance as bottom pulled up.	legs straight - no resistance	knee flexes - remains flexed when bottom lifts up	flexion stays when back+bottom lifts up	

Head and trunk control

HEAD CONTROL (1) *(extensor tone)* Infant sitting upright. Encircle chest with both hands holding shoulders. Let head drop forward.	no attempt to raise head	raises head: remains vertical, wobbles	head cannot be flexed	
HEAD CONTROL (2) *(flexor tone)* Infant sitting upright. Encircle chest with both hands holding shoulders. Let head drop backward.	no attempt to raise head	raises head: remains vertical, wobbles		
HEAD LAG Pull infant to sit by both wrists & support head slightly.	head drops back & stays	lifts head in line with body		
VENTRAL SUSPENSION Hold infant horizontally under the abdomen. Look at position of back, arms, and limbs. If it looks different - DRAW!	back curved, head & limbs hang straight	back straight, head in line or above body		

Other signs

BODY MOVEMENTS Observe during the examination when the infant is awake and quiet.	absent or Infrequent	mainly smooth, alternating	cramped, athetoid, jerky, or other abnormal movements. (Describe)	
TREMORS AND STARTLES	none	only occasional	tremulous *always*, many startles	
MORO REFLEX Put infant in position shown in diagram. Bring head forward, and suddenly let it go back slightly.	no response; or full abduction of the arms, extension at the elbow; no adduction	full abduction, followed by adduction	• minimal adduction or abduction •difficult to elicit	
AUDITORY ORIENTATION Ability to respond to rattle. Rattle 5 inches (12.5 cm) from ear.	no response	brightens, turns to stimulus either side		
VISUAL ORIENTATION Ability to track red ball or target.	no focusing. Tracking < 60	good horizontal and vertical tracking		
ALERTNESS Response to visual stimulation	when awake variable response to orientation	alertness sustained, may use stimulus to come to alert state		

Abnormal signs	Suck		Facial palsy		Abnormal eye movements		Sunset sign		Fisted hand		Clonus	
	Y	N	Y	N	Y	N	Y	N	Y	N	Y	N

NB: Infants with 2 or more items in blocked-and-shaded areas need to be reassessed.

138

common in such countries, early discharge of the affected infants is still highly desirable, partly for medical and partly for economic reasons. Cross-infection, particularly in over-crowded hospitals, is a threat to both mothers and infants. Prolonged hospitalization also puts financial burdens both on the health care services and on the parents. However, as asphyxiated infants are undoubtedly at a heightened risk of early death, a routine evaluation that could select on clinical grounds the infants who are essentially neurologically intact, and therefore at least risk, would be extremely helpful.

A widely and easily applicable neonatal neurological examination is also needed in many research settings. A prime example is that of areas in which malaria is endemic, where one wishes to study the effect on the newborn infant of maternal malaria or of antimalarial drugs given to the mother. While there is a great need to evaluate infants born in these areas, trained medical and even paramedical staff are usually in short supply. One challenge we have had in recent years was a request from such areas to devise an examination that could be taught to staff, such as traditional midwives, who are experienced in handling newborn infants but who have had no medical training and whose literacy may be limited.

Many of the personnel we trained, in several developing countries, had some experience in looking for tone patterns, as they were often familiar with methods of assessing gestational age. We found it relatively easy to teach all the items assessing tone in our original neurological proforma. Two adaptations were essential. The stick figures on the proforma had to be enlarged, as the examiners relied heavily on them, and both their visual acuity and the ambient lighting was often less than optimal. The text, in particular the instructions, had to be put into more colloquial language. Items such as head raising in the prone, arm release in the prone, and the defensive reaction had to be omitted, as both the examiners and the mothers found them frightening. The items relating to abnormal movements and postures were simplified. The observers generally had difficulty categorizing movements, in particular any abnormal movements such as mouthing, jerky or athetoid movement, and abnormal eye movements. As the interobserver reliability on these items was poor, they were omitted. We also omitted tendon reflexes, as the examiners found them difficult and thus never recorded them. The test for the sucking reflex was modified, as the introduction of anything but the mother's nipple into the infant's mouth was thought to be highly undesirable in places where hand-washing facilities are limited. We asked the examiners instead to watch the infant feeding on the breast. The three items describing the infants' behaviour, "peak of excitement", "irritability", and "consolability," were redefined and condensed in two items.

A proforma designed for research related to maternal malaria on the Thai–Burmese border is illustrated in Figure 7.2. The personnel taking part in the project, who were trained by one of the medical research staff to perform the testing, were mainly traditional midwives,

Fig. 7.1 *(facing page)*. Neurological screening tests for general use in term infants. The proforma tries to designate the optimal response for each item and the obviously abnormal ones. Borderline responses have been omitted but can be commented on.

HAMMERSMITH SHORT NEONATAL NEUROLOGICAL EXAMINATION

NAME:_____, CODE:_____, No. OF EXAM:_____,

D.O.B.:_____, D.O.E.:_____, AGE:_____, G.A.:_____, SEX:_____,BW:_____,

						S T A T E	A S Y M E T
POSTURE Baby lying on back. Look mainly at position of the legs, but also note arms. You may change drawing.	arms & legs extended	legs slightly flexed	legs well flexed but not adducted	legs well flexed & adducted near belly	arms very flexed, legs very extended		
ARM RECOIL Quickly extend (straighten) both arms; put next to body. Count to two. Let go. Repeat 3 times.	arm does not flex	arm flexes slowly, not always, not completely	arm flexes slowly, more completely	arm flexes and remains flexed	arm difficult to extend; snap back forcefully		
ARM TRACTION Hold wrist and pull upward. Note flexion at arm, and resistance while shoulder lifts off table.	arm remains straight - no resistance	arm flexes slightly or some resistance felt	arm flexes well till shoulder lifts, then straightens	arm flexes and remains flexed as shoulder lifts	arm remains flexed when body lifts up		
LEG RECOIL Take both ankles, bend hips+knee. Quickly extend when infant not pushing. Let go. Repeat X 3	No flexion	incomplete flexion, not every time	complete slow flexion	complete fast flexion	legs difficult to extend; snap back forcefully		
LEG TRACTION Hold ankle, pull leg upwards. Look at flexion & resistance as bottom pulled up.	leg straight - no resistance	leg flexes slightly or some resistance felt	leg flexes well till bottom lifts up	knee flexes - remains flexed when bottom up	flexion stays when back+bottom up		
POPLITEAL ANGLE Fix knee on abdomen (belly), try to extend knee with first finger. Note distance (angle) between upper and lower limb.	180°	≈150°	≈110°	≈90°	<90°		
HEAD CONTROL (1) Baby sitting upright. Encircle chest with both hands holding shoulders. Let head drop forward.	no attempt to raise head	infant tries: effort better felt than seen	raises head but drops forward or back	raises head: remains vertical, wobbles			
HEAD CONTROL (2) Baby sitting upright. Encircle chest with both hands holding shoulders. Let head drop backward.	no attempt to raise head	infant tries: effort better felt than seen	raises head but drops forward or back	raises head: remains vertical, wobbles	head upright or extended; cannot be passively flexed (pushed forward)		
HEAD LAG Pull baby to sit by the wrists & support head slightly.	head drops & stays back	tries to lift head but it drops back	able to lift head slightly	lifts head in line with body	head in front of body		
VENTRAL SUSPENSION Hold baby horizontal under the belly. Look at posture of back, arms, legs, and head. If it looks different, DRAW!	back curved, head & limbs hang straight	back curved, head ↓, limb slightly flexed	back slightly curved, limbs flexed	back straight, head in line with body, limbs flexed	back straight, head above body		

140

MOVEMENTS						STATE	ASYMM
SPONTANEOUS MOVEMENT Watch baby while (s)he is lying on back.	no movement	few stretches, no other movement	jerky movement, stretches, but also some smooth movement	smooth movements of arms + legs	fits, cramped or other abnormal movements: DESCRIBE!!		
ABNORMAL HAND OR TOE POSTURES	hands open	hands fisted or thumbs adduct intermittently but open	hands fist or thumb adducts, or finger & thumb oppose	big toe up (extended) or all toes flex			
TREMOR	no tremor	tremor only when crying or after Moro reflex	some tremor when awake	frequent tremors	continuous tremors		
STARTLE Similar movements to Moro reflex but not doing Moro test	no startle	startle to sudden noise or bang on table	2 or 3 spontaneous startles	3 - 5 spontaneous startles	more than 6 spontaneous startles		

REFLEXES = test both sides

SUCK & GAG Watch on breast; if no suck is seen, put little finger into mouth with pulp of finger upwards.	no gag / no suck	weak suck only: (a) irregular (b) regular No stripping	infant sucks well on the breast	strong suck: (a) irregular (b) regular Good stripping	no suck but strong clenching		
PALMAR GRASP Stroke inside of hand. DO NOT TOUCH BACK OF HAND!!	no reaction	short, weak flexion of fingers	strong flexion of fingers	strong finger flexion, shoulder ↑	strong finger flexion, whole body ↑		
PLANTAR GRASP Press on sole below toes.	no response	toes flex (bend) slightly	toes curve around finger				
MORO REFLEX Put baby in position shown in drawing 1 below. Bring head forward and suddenly let it fall back slightly.	no response	full abduction of the arms, extension at the elbow, no adduction	full abduction, little or delayed adduction	arms do not fully abduct but good adduction	• adduction only • extension at the elbow only		
PLACING Hold infant upright. Stroke front of the baby's lower leg on edge of table.	nothing happens	baby flexes ankle	baby flexes hip, knee, and ankle & steps on table				

ORIENTATION AND BEHAVIOUR

EYES	does not open eyes	normal eye movement, eyes move together	abnormal eye movements: DESCRIBE!!				
AUDITORY ORIENTATION Must be asleep. Wrap infant. Hold rattle 10-15 cm (4-6 inches) from ear.	no reaction	brightens (wakes up)	turns eyes and sometimes turns head a bit also	turns eyes and head fully to side of noise	turns head and eyes strongly to noise; does not tire		
VISUAL ALERTNESS Wrap infant, wake up with rattle if needed or rock baby a bit. Look if baby can see and follow red ball (R) or a target (T).	does not follow or focus on red ball or target	stills, focuses, follows very briefly to side and up but loses it quickly	follows with eyes to the side and up, may turn head	follows with eyes to the side and up; turns head always	follows in a circle		
	R T	R T	R T	R T	R T		
ALERTNESS Tested as response to red ball (R) or target (T). How long infant interested.	will not respond to red ball	when awake, looks only briefly	when awake, looks at red ball but loses it	keeps interest in red ball	does not tire		
	R T	R T	R T	R T	R T		
PEAK OF EXCITEMENT Circle "H" if high-pitch cry	quiet all the time	awakes briefly, does not cry	awakes briefly, cries sometimes	cries always when handled	cries always		
	H	H	H	H	H		
CONSOLABILITY How easy is it to make baby quiet?	never awake or crying	awake but never cries, consoling not needed	becomes quiet when talked to	needs picking up to console	cannot be consoled		

COMMENT: EXAMINER:

Fig. 7.2 *(above and on facing page)*. Proforma adapted for a study of newborn infants on the Thai–Burmese border whose mothers had malaria or had been treated with antimalarial drugs. Infants with two or more items in the blocked-and-shaded areas need to be reassessed.

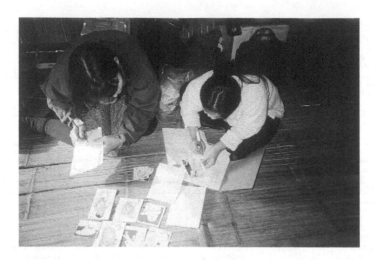

Fig. 7.3. Neurological examination in a developing country: learning to score.

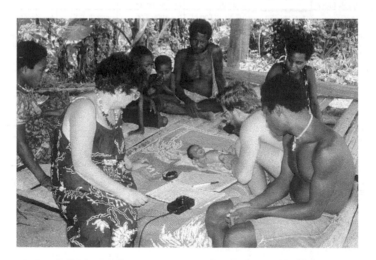

Fig. 7.4. Neurological examination in a village in Papua New Guinea.

and there were some additional medically untrained staff who were recruited entirely for this project (Figs. 7.3, 7.4). The trainees achieved a very high interobserver reliability between themselves and the medical person who trained them, but more frequent checks were needed to maintain this reliability than would be needed with medically trained personnel. This led to some interesting problems. In the area in question, approximately 700 infants were delivered per year: most of these deliveries took place in a room set aside for this purpose at the unit, but a significant proportion of the mothers still delivered at home

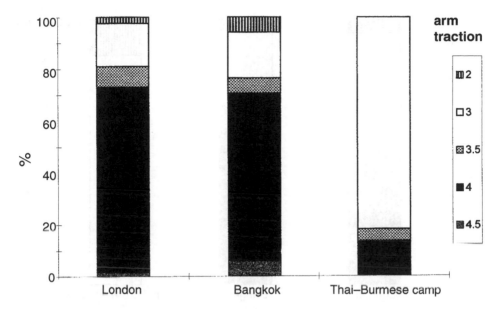

Fig. 7.5. Scores on the arm traction test in three separate cohorts of term infants, from London, Bangkok, and a refugee camp on the Thai– Burmese border. Note that while sustained arm flexion (score 3.5 or 4) was achieved in approximately 80% of infants in London and Bangkok, only 20% of the infants in the refugee camp achieved this score.

in their own huts, often quite far away from the main unit. All home deliveries were also assessed by the staff. Initially, there were 6 or 7 examiners to cover the distance. This, however, meant that some of the testers examined only a few newborn infants a year and thus lost their skills. The number of examiners was therefore cut, greatly increasing their reliability.

The new proforma has now been in use for over 3 years, to assess more than a thousand infants. The data for this cohort have not yet been fully analysed, but some interesting preliminary findings have already emerged. The data from a pilot study of the infants examined in the refugee camp on the Thai–Burmese border have been compared with data collected in a large maternity hospital in Bangkok and in a large maternity hospital in London. While for some of the items there were apparently no differences, or only minor ones, between the three cohorts, striking differences could be observed in some of the items assessing tone and in those assessing tremor and visual orientation. These are illustrated in Figures 7.5–7.8.

As the findings for the Bangkok cohort and the (white) London infants were similar to each other but differed from those for the infants in the refugee camp, the differences are less likely to be due to ethnic differences than to more specific problems relating to the camp, such as the nutritional state of the mother.

143

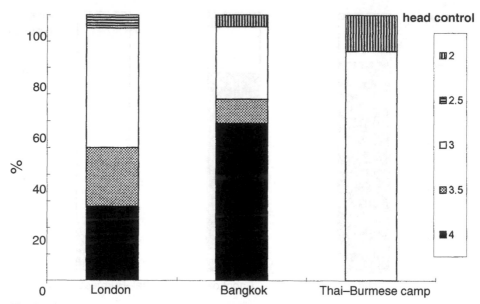

Fig. 7.6. Scores on the test for head control in the same cohorts of term infants as in Figure 7.3. Note that while the London and Bangkok cohorts did differ in the proportion of infants who could hold their head upright (scores 3.5 and 4), none of the infants in the refugee camp could do so.

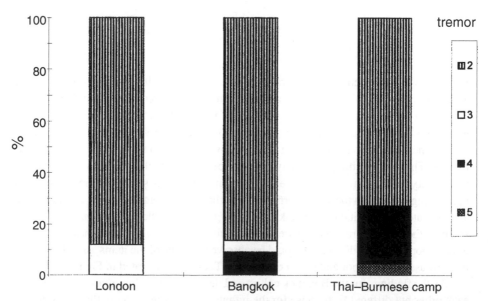

Fig. 7.7. Scores for tremor in the same cohorts of term infants as in Figure 7.3. Note that while none of the London infants and only 10% of the Bangkok infants showed marked tremor, this was found in approximately 25% of the infants in the refugee camp.

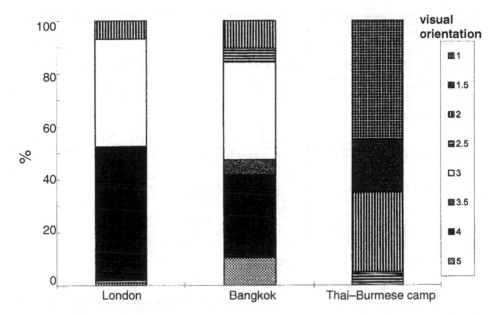

Fig. 7.8. Scores for visual orientation in the same cohorts of term infants as in Figure 7.3. Note that while visual tracking (scores 3 and 4) was present in approximately 90% of both London and Bangkok infants, none of the infants in the refugee camp achieved these scores.

This proforma has also been piloted in several studies in maternal malaria in Africa. Here all the infants were delivered in a hospital and most patients were discharged within 6 hours. All the infants had to have an assessment of gestational age and possibly a neurological examination before discharge. Thus, enough examiners had to be trained to cover shifts and absences, but without necessarily giving each examiner a large number of infants. To increase their experience and interobserver reliability, the examiners therefore worked in pairs. During the pilot study, they were able to pick out a number of infants who were very quiet, who looked very alert but showed poor visual orientation, whose head control was always suboptimal, and who frequently were tremulous. All these infants were found to have hypoglycaemia.

Because the African examiners were under pressure to discharge the patients in time to let them reach home before dark, even the examination used in Thailand proved to be too long, and the proformas were often left uncompleted. To meet such pressures but still achieve full recording of the items of greatest interest in this cohort, we cut the time of the examination even further by leaving in only the items most essential for their needs. We also excluded from the separate neurological proforma items that were tested already during the assessment of gestational age. The resulting simplified proforma is shown in Figure 7.9.

ARM TRACTION Hold wrist and pull up. Note flexion at arm and resistance while shoulder lifts off table.	arm remains straight - no resistance	arm flexes slightly or some resistance	arm flexes well till shoulder lifts	arm flexes and remains flexed	arm remains flexed when body lifts up
LEG TRACTION Hold ankle, pull leg upwards. Look at flexion & resistance as bottom is pulled up.	leg straight - no resistance	leg flexes slightly or some resistance	leg flexes well till bottom lifts up	knee flexes, stays flexed when bottom up	flexion stays when back + bottom up
HEAD CONTROL (1) Infant sitting. Hold at shoulder. Let head drop forward.	no attempt to raise head	infant tries: effort better felt than seen	raises head but drops forward or back	raises head: remains vertical, wobbles	
HEAD CONTROL (2) Infant sitting. Hold at shoulder. Let head drop backward.	no attempt to raise head	infant tries: effort better felt than seen	raises head but drops forward or back	raises head: remains vertical, wobbles	
ABNORMAL HAND OR TOE POSTURES		open hands	hands fisted or thumb adducted but opens	hands fisted or thumb adducted all the time	big toe up (extended) all the time
TREMOR		no tremor	tremor only when crying	some tremor or startles when awake	lot of tremor when awake
VISUAL ORIENTATION Wrap infant, wake up with rattle if needed or rock baby a bit. Look if baby can see and follow red ball or target	does not follow or focus on 1) red ball 2) target	focuses, follows briefly to side and up but quickly loses 1) red ball 2) target	follows with eyes horizontally and vertically 1) red ball 2) target	always follows with eyes to the side and up may turn head 1) red ball 2) target	follows in a circle, does not tire 1) red ball 2) target
AUDITORY ORIENTATION Must not be asleep. Wrap infant. Hold rattle 10-15 cm (4-6 inches) from ear.	no reaction	brightens (wakes up)	turns eyes and sometimes turns head a bit also	turned eyes and head fully to side of noise	turns head and eyes jerkily to noise *always*, does not tire
PEAK OF EXCITEMENT	quiet all the time	awakes briefly, does not cry	awakes briefly, cries sometimes, easily consolable	cries when handled	cries always, unconsolable
SUCK & GAG Watch on breast; if no suck is seen, put little finger into mouth with pulp of finger upwards.	no gag / no suck	weak suck only: (a) irregular (b) regular No stripping	infant sucks well on the breast	strong suck: (a) irregular (b) regular Good stripping	no suck but strong clenching

Fig. 7.9. Short proforma to be integrated with the assessment-of-gestation form to achieve rapid recording of tone, jitteriness, and alertness. Infants with 2 or more items in the blocked-and-shaded areas need to be reassessed

146

Proforma for neurological examination after the neonatal period

We applied the principles of the neonatal neurological examination to a proforma (the Hammersmith Infant Neurological Examination) for use as a standard neurological examination after the neonatal period (Fig. 7.10). The aim was again to have some instructions for the examination incorporated in the sheet and to score the items with the help of diagrams. As this proforma was intended for use from the end of the first month until just under 2 years of age, we separated the age-dependent from the non-age-dependent items.

The first section consists of 26 non-age-dependent items assessing cranial nerve function, posture, movements, tone, and reflexes. This section was designed in accordance with the frequency distribution of the neurological findings in a cohort of 92 twelve-month-old infants and 43 eighteen-month-old infants who had no known perinatal risk factors. The findings in column 1 are the ones most frequently seen in the normal population (75% or more), those in column 2 are seen less frequently (in 25% or fewer) but in more than 10% of normal infants, and the findings in columns 3 and 4 are seen in only 10% or fewer of normal infants. Each item is scored individually, and a global score can be obtained by summing all the scores for the individual items.

The second section includes a few selected motor items, in which normality and abnormality are age dependent. This section provides a summary of motor milestones and gives the opportunity, when the children are seen at later age, to record the age at which the various milestones are reached.

We also added more items, adapted from the Bayley scales, to assess the infant's behavioural state, because this can affect the outcome of the examination.

This proforma has been used in a population of infants with HIE. The preliminary results suggest that while infants with grade-I HIE, either with normal MRI or with minimal changes, have scores similar to those for a normal population, the infants with grade-II HIE have more variable scores, depending mainly on the presence and severity of the lesions and in particular on the severity of basal ganglia involvement.

The items included in this version of the proforma are the ones that we found most useful and that showed good interobserver reliability even in inexperienced staff. It could be easily adapted for individual needs, by including other items that might be needed for specific research projects.

HAMMERSMITH INFANT NEUROLOGICAL EXAMINATION

Name: **Date of birth:**

Gestational age: **Date of examination:**

SUMMARY OF EXAMINATION

No of asymmetries in section 1:

Neurological items score:

Behavioural score:

COMMENTS:

Cranial nerves functions

Posture

Movements

Tone

Reflexes and reactions

Behaviour

SECTION 1 : NEUROLOGICAL ITEMS

Assessment of cranial nerve function

	column 1 (score 2)	c. 2 (sc. 1.5)	column 3 (score 1)	column 4 (score 0)	A	comment
Facial appearance (at rest and when crying or stimulated)	smiles or reacts to stimuli by closing eyes and grimacing		closes eyes but not tightly; poor facial expression	expressionless; does not react to stimuli		
Eye appearance	normal conjugated eye movements		**intermittent** deviation of eyes or abnormal movements	**continuous** deviation of eyes or abnormal movements		
Auditory response test the response to rattle or bell	reacts to stimuli on both sides		doubtful reaction to stimuli or asymmetrical	does not react to stimuli		
Visual response test the ability to follow a red ball or moving object	follows the object for a complete arc		follows the object for an incomplete arc, or asymmetry	does not follow the object		
Sucking/swallowing watch the infant suck on breast or bottle	good suck and swallowing		poor suck and/or swallowing	no sucking reflex, no swallowing		

Fig. 7.10 *(above, and next 3 pages)* The Hammersmith Infant Neurological Examination: a neurological examination for infants after the neonatal period (from 1 month to 24 months of age).

	column 1 (score 2)	c 2 (sc.1.5)	column 3 (score 1)	column 4 (score 0)	A	
Head in sitting	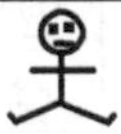 straight; in midline		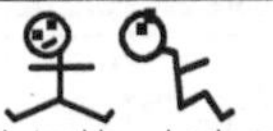 slightly to side *or* backward *or* forward	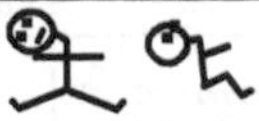 markedly to side *or* backward *or* forward		
Trunk in sitting	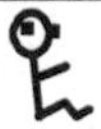 straight		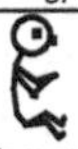 slightly curved or bent to side	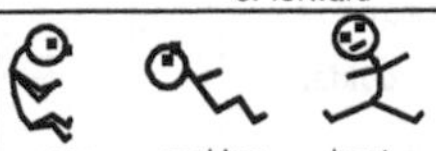 very rounded / rocking back / bent sideways		
Arms at rest	in neutral position: central, straight *or* slightly bent		**slight** internal rotation *or* external rotation	**marked** internal rotation *or* external rotation or dystonic posture hemiplegic posture		
Hands	hands open		**intermittent** adducted thumb *or* fisting	**persistent** adducted thumb *or* fisting		
Legs In sitting	able to sit with straight back, and legs straight or slightly bent (long sitting)		sit with straight back but knees bent at 15-20 °	unable to sit straight unless knees markedly bent (no long sitting)		
in supine and in standing	legs in neutral position: straight *or* slightly bent	**slight** internal rotation or external rotation	internal rotation *or* external rotation at hips	**marked** internal rotation *or* external rotation or fixed extension or flexion or contractures at hips and knees		
Feet in supine and in standing	central; in neutral position		**slight** internal rotation *or* external rotation	**marked** internal rotation *or* external rotation at the ankle		
			intermittent tendency to stand on tiptoes; *or* toes up or curling under	**persistent** tendency to stand on tiptoes *or* toes up or curling under		
	toes straight midway between flexion and extension					

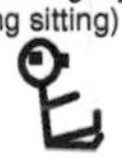

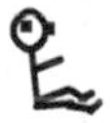

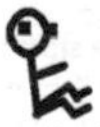

Movements

	column 1 (score 2)	c 2 (sc.1.5)	column 3 (score 1)	column 4 (score 0)	A	
Quantity watch infant lying in the supine	normal		excessive or sluggish	minimal or none		
Quality	free, alternating, smooth		jerky, slight tremor	• cramped & synchronous • extensor spasms • athetoid • ataxic • very tremulous • myoclonic spasm • dystonic		

Fig. 7.10 *(continued)*

149

Tone

	column 1 (score 2) Range:	c. 2 (sc.1.5)	column 3 (score 1)	column 4 (score 0)	A
Scarf sign Take the infant's hand and pull the arm across the chest until there is resistance. Note the position of the elbow.	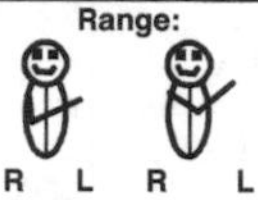 R L R L		R L	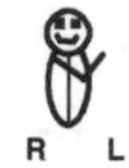 R L R L or	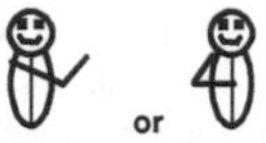
Passive shoulder elevation Lift arm next to the infant's head. Note resistance at shoulder and elbow.	resistance, but overcome 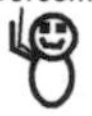 R L		no resistance 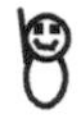 R L	resistance, not overcome 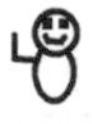 R L	
Pronation/supination Steady upper arm while pronating and supinating forearm. Note resistance.	full pronation and supination, no resistance,		full pronation and supination but resistance to be overcome	full pronation and supination not possible, marked resistance	
Adductors With the infant's legs extended, open them as far as possible. The angle formed by the legs is noted.	Range: 150°-80° 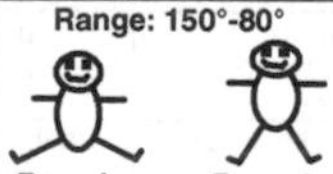 R L R L	150°-160° 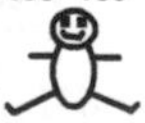 R L	>170° 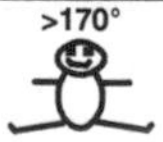 R L	< 80° R L	
Popliteal angle Legs are flexed at the hip simultaneously on to the side of the abdomen, then extended at the knee until there is resistance. Note angle between lower and upper leg.	Range: 150°-110° 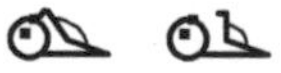 R L R L	150°-160° 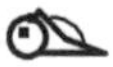 R L	~90° or > 170° 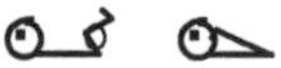 R L R L	<80° R L	
Ankle dorsiflexion With knee extended, dorsiflex ankle. Note the angle between foot and leg.	Range: 30°-85° 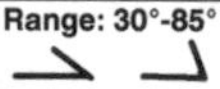 R L R L	20°-30° R L	< 20°or 90° R L R L	> 90° R L	
Pulled to sit Pull infant to sit by wrists. 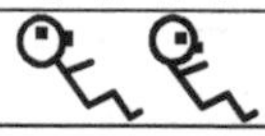 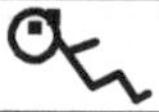 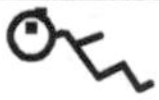					
Ventral suspension Hold infant in ventral suspension; note position of back, limbs, and head. 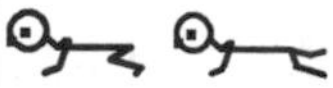 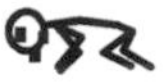 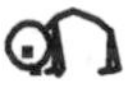					

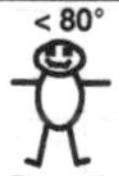

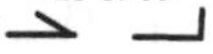

Reflexes and reactions

Tendon Reflexes	easily elicitable biceps knee ankle	mildly brisk bic knee ank	brisk biceps knee ankle	clonus or absent biceps knee ankle		
Arm protection Pull the infant by one arm from the supine position and note the reaction of the opposite side.	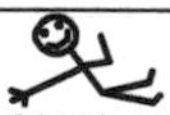 arm & hand extend R L		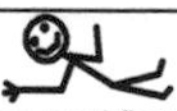 arm semi-flexed R L	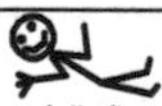 arm fully flexed R L		
Vertical suspension Hold infant under axilla. Make sure legs do not touch any surface.	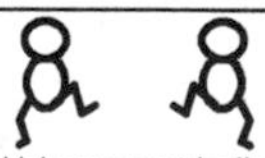 kicks symmetrically		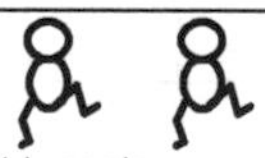 kicks one leg more, or poor kicking	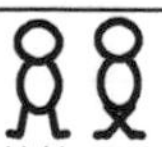 no kicking even if stimulated, or scissoring		
Lateral tilting (describe side up). Infant held vertically, tilt quickly to horizontal. Note spine, limbs, and head.	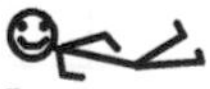 R L	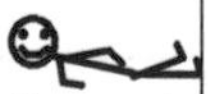 R L	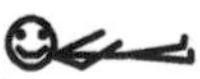 R L	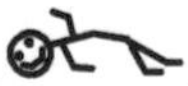 R L		
Forward parachute Infant held vertically and suddenly tilted forward. Note reaction of the arms.	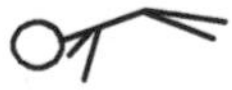 (after 6 months)		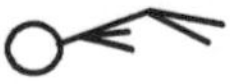 (after 6 months)			

Fig. 7.10 *(continued)*

SECTION 2: MOTOR MILESTONES

Head control	unable to maintain head upright (normal < 3 mo)	wobbles (normal at 4 mo)	all the time maintained upright (normal at 5 mo)			
Sitting	cannot sit	sits with support at hips (normal at 4 mo)	props (normal at 6 mo)	stable sit (normal at 7-8 mo)	pivots (rotates) (normal at 9 mo)	Observed: Reported (age):
Voluntary grasp	no grasp	uses whole hand	index finger and thumb but immature grasp	pincer grasp		Observed: Reported (age):
Ability to kick (in supine)	no kicking	kicks horizontally legs do not lift	upward (vertically) (normal at 3 mo)	touches leg (normal at 4-5 mo)	touches toes (normal at 5-6 mo)	Observed: Reported (age):
Rolling	no rolling	rolling to side (normal at 4 mo)	prone to supine (normal at mo)	supine to prone (normal at mo)		Observed: Reported (age):
Crawling	does not lift head	on elbow (normal at 3 mo)	on outstretched hand (normal at 4 mo)	crawling flat on abdomen (normal at 8 mo)	crawling on hands and knees (normal at 10 mo)	Observed: Reported (age):
Standing	does not support weight	supports weight (normal at 4 mo)	stands with support (normal at 7 mo)	stands unaided (normal at 12 mo)		Observed: Reported (age):
Walking		bouncing (normal at 6 mo)	cruising (walks holding on) (normal at 12 mo)	walking independently (normal at 15 mo)		Observed: Reported (age):

SECTION 3: BEHAVIOUR

	1	2	3	4	5	6	Comment
State of consciousness	unrousable	drowsy	sleepy but wakes easily	awake but no interest	loses interest	maintains interest	
Emotional state	irritable, not consolable	irritable, mother can console	irritable when approached	neither happy or unhappy	happy, smiling		
Social orientation	avoiding, withdrawn	hesitant	accepts approach	friendly			

Score for behaviour:

Fig. 7.10 *(continued)*

151

REFERENCES

Als H, Tronick F, Adamson L, Brazelton T B. (1976) The behaviour of the full-term but underweight newborn infant. *Developmental Medicine and Child Neurology* **18:** 590–602.

Amiel-Tison C. (1979) Birth injury as a cause of brain dysfunction in full term newborns. In: Korobkin R, Guilleminault C, editors. *Advances in Perinatal Neurology.* SP Medical and Scientific Books. p 57–83.

— Grenier A. (1980) *Évaluation neurologique du nouveau-né et du nourisson.* Paris: Masson.

— Korobkin R, Esque-Vaucouloux M T. (1977) Neck extensor hypertonia: a clinical sign of insult to the central nervous system of the newborn. *Early Human Development* **1:** 181–190.

— Barrier G, Shnider S M, et al. (1982) A new neurologic and adaptive capacity scoring system for evaluating obstetric medications in full term newborn infants. *Anesthesiology* **56:** 340–350.

André-Thomas, de Ajuriaguerra J. (1949) *Étude sémiologique du tonus musculaire.* Paris: Éditions Médicales Flammarion.

— Saint-Anne Dargassies S. (1952) *Études neurologiques sur le nouveau-né et la jeune nourisson.* Paris: Masson.

— Chesni Y, Saint-Anne Dargassies S. (1960) *The Neurological Examination of the Infant.* Clinics in Developmental Medicine No. 1. London: National Spastics Society.

Banker BQ, Larroche JC. (1962) Periventricular leukomalacia in neonates: complications and sequelae. *Archives of Neurology* **7:** 386–410.

Beintema D. (1968) *A Neurological Study of Newborn Infants.* Clinics in Developmental Medicine No. 28. London: William Heinemann Medical Books.

Brazelton TB. (1973) *Neonatal Behavioral Assessment Scale.* Clinics in Developmental Medicine No. 50. London: Spastics International Medical Publications/William Heinemann Medical Books; Philadelphia: J B Lippincott Co.

— Nugent JK. (1995) *Neonatal Behavioural Assessment Scale.* 3rd edition. Clinics in Developmental Medicine No. 137. London: Mac Keith Press.

— Tronick E, Lechtig A, et al. (1977) The behavior of nutritionally deprived Guatemalan infants. *Developmental Medicine and Child Neurology* **19:** 364–372.

Casaer P, Daniels H, Devlieger H, et al. (1982) Feeding behaviour in preterm neonates. *Early Human Development* **7:** 331–346.

Cioni G, Prechtl HFR. (1990) Preterm and early post-term motor behaviour in low-risk premature infants. *Early Human Development* **23:**159–193.

— Ferrari F, Einspieler C, et al. (1997) Comparison between observation of spontaneous movements and neurological examination in preterm infants. *Journal of Pediatrics* **130:** 704–711.

de Vries LS, Dubowitz LMS, Dubowitz V, et al. (1985) Predictive value of cranial ultrasound in the newborn baby: a reappraisal. *Lancet* **ii:** 137–140.

— Heckmatt J Z, Burrin JM, et al. (1986) Low serum thyroxine concentrations and neural maturation in preterm infants. *Archives of Disease in Childhood* **61:** 862–866.

—Dubowitz LMS, Pennock J, Dubowitz V. (1990) *Brain Disorder in the Newborn.* London: Wolfe Medical Publications.

— Eken P, Dubowitz LMS. (1992) The spectrum of leukomalacia using cranial ultrasound. *Behavioural Brain Research* **49:** 1–6.

— Groenendaal F, Eken P, et al. (1997) Infarcts in the vascular distribution of the middle cerebral artery in preterm and fullterm infants. *Neuropediatrics* **28:** 88–96.

Donovan DE, Coves P, Paine RS. (1962) The prognostic implications of neurological abnormalities in the neonatal period. *Neurology* **12:** 910–914.

Dubowitz LMS. (1985) Neurological assessment of the full term and preterm newborn infant. In: Hare LS, Anastolsiow NY, editors. *The At-risk Infant: Psychosocial Medical Aspects.* Baltimore: Paul H Brooks. p 185–196.

— Dubowitz V. (1977) *Gestational Age of the Newborn: A Clinical Manual.* Reading, MA; Menlo Park, CA; London, UK; etc: Addison-Wesley.

— — (1981) *The Neurological Assessment of the Preterm and Full-term Newborn Infant.* Clinics in Developmental Medicine No. 79. London: Spastics International Medical Publications/William Heinemann Medical Books.

— — Goldberg C. (1970) Clinical assessment of gestational age in the newborn infant. *Journal of Pediatrics* **77:** 1–10.

— — Morante A, Verghote M. (1980) Visual function in the premature and fullterm newborn infant. *Developmental Medicine and Child Neurology* **22:** 465–475.

— Levene MI, Morante A, et al. (1981) Neurological signs in neonatal intraventricular hemorrhage: correlation with real-time ultrasound. *Journal of Pediatrics* **99:** 127–133.

— Dubowitz V, Goldberg C. (1983) Comparison of neurological function in growth-retarded and appropriate sized full-term newborn infants in two ethnic groups. *South African Medical Journal* **61:** 1003–1007.

— — Paimer PG, et al. (1984) Correlation of neurologic assessment in the preterm newborn infant with outcome at one year. *Journal of Pediatrics* **105:** 452–456.

— Mushin J, de Vries L, Arden GB. (1986) Visual function in the newborn infant: is it cortically mediated? *Lancet* **i:** 1139–1140.

— Mercuri E, Dubowitz V. (1998) An optimality score for the neurological examination of the full-term newborn. *Journal of Pediatrics* **133:** 406–416.

Eken P, de Vries LS, van der Graaf Y, et al. (1995) Haemorrhagic–ischaemic lesions of the neonatal brain: correlation between cerebral visual impairment, neurodevelopmental outcome and MRI in infancy. *Developmental Medicine and Child Neurology* **37:** 41–55.

— — van Nieuwenhuizen O, et al. (1996) Early predictors of cerebral visual impairment in infants with cystic leukomalacia. *Neuropediatrics* **27:** 16–25.

Eyler FD, Carter RC, Resnick HB. (1986) Dubowitz Neurological assessment of preterm infants: an update. *Pediatric Research* **20(4):** A377.

— — — Eitzman DV. (1987) Dubowitz Neurological assessment of preterm infants: developmental outcome. *Pediatric Research* **21(4):** A394.

— Delgado-Hackey M, Woods NS, Carter RL. (1991) Quantification of the Dubowitz Neurological assessment of preterm neonates: developmental outcome. *Infant Behavioural Development* **14:** 445–469.

Farr V, Mitchell RG, Neligan GA, Parkin JM. (1966) The definition of some external characteristics used in the assessment of gestational age in the newborn infant. *Developmental Medicine and Child Neurology* **8:** 507–511.

Govaert P, de Vries LS. (1997) *An Atlas of Neonatal Brain Sonography.* Clinics in Developmental Medicine Nos. 141–142. London: Mac Keith Press.

Graham FK. (1956) *Behavioural Differences Between Normal and Traumatized Newborns. I. The Test Procedures.* Psychological Monographs **70:** 1–16.

— Matarazzo RG, Caldwell BM. (1956) *Behavioural Differences Between Normal and Traumatized Newborns: II. Standardization, Reliability and Validity.* Psychological Monographs **70:** 127–28.

Haataja L, Mercuri E, Regev R, et al. (1999) Optimality score for the neurological examination of the infant at 12 and 18 months of age. *Journal of Pediatrics* **135:** 153–161.

Howard J, Parmelee AH, Kopp CB, Littman B. (1976) A neurological comparison of preterm and full term infants at term conceptual age. *Journal of Pediatrics* **88:** 995–1002.

Illingworth RS. (1980) *The Development of the Infant and Young Child.* Edinburgh: Churchill Livingstone.

Jongmans M, Henderson S, de Vries L, Dubowitz L. (1993) Duration of periventricular densities in preterm infants and neurological outcome at 6 years. *Archives of Disease in Childhood* **69:** 9–13.

— Mercuri E, de Vries L, et al. (1997) Minor neurological signs and perceptual motor difficulties in prematurely born children. *Archives of Disease in Childhood* **76:** F9–F14.

Kurtzberg D, Vaughan HG Jr, Daum C, et al. (1979) Neurobehavioural performance of low-birthweight infants at 40 weeks conceptional age: comparison with normal fullterm infants. *Developmental Medicine Child Neurology* **21:** 590–597.

Lacey JL, Henderson-Smart DJ, Edwards DA, Storey B. (1985) The early development of head control in preterm infants. *Early Human Development* **11:** 199–212.

Leijon I, Finnstrom 0. (1982) Correlation between neurological examination and behavioural assessment of the newborn infant. *Early Human Development* **7:** 119–130.

Levene MI, Wigglesworth JS, Dubowitz V. (1981) Cerebral structure and intraventricular haemorrhage in the neonate: a real time ultrasound study. *Archives of Disease in Childhood* **56:** 416–424.

153

Mac Keith R. (1977) In: Prechtl HFR. *The Neurological Examination of the Full term Newborn Infant*. 2nd ed. Clinics in Developmental Medicine No. 63. London: Spastics International Medical Publications/William Heinemann Medical Books. Preface, p v.

Mercuri E, Dubowitz LMS. (1996) The prognosis of neonatal neurological abnormalities. *Baillère's Clinical Paediatrics* **4**: 393–408.

— Cowan F, Rutherford M, et al. (1995) Ischaemic and haemorrhagic brain lesions in newborns with seizures and normal Apgar scores. *Archives of Disease in Childhood* **73**: F67–F74.

— Atkinson J, Braddick O, et al. (1997) Basal ganglia damage and impaired visual function in the newborn infant. *Archives of Disease in Childhood* **77**: F111–F114.

— Rutherford M, Cowan F, et al. (1999a) Early prognostic indicators of outcome in infants with neonatal cerebral infarction: a clinical, EEG and MRI study. *Pediatrics* **103**: 31–38.

— Guzzetta A, Haataja L, et al. (1999b) Neonatal neurological examination in infants with hypoxic ischaemic encephalopathy: correlation with MRI findings. *Neuropediatrics* **30**: 83–89.

Molteno C, Grosz P, Wallace P, Jones M. (1995) Neurological examination of the preterm and full-term infant at risk for developmental disabilities using the Dubowitz Neurological assessment. *Early Human Development* **41**: 167–176.

Palmer PG, Dubowitz LMS, Verghote M, Dubowitz V. (1982) Neurological and ncurobehavioural differences between preterm infants at term and full term newborn infants. *Neuropediatrics* **13**: 183–189.

Pape KE, Wigglesworth JS. (1979) *Haemorrhage, Ischemia and the Perinatal Brain*. Clinics in Developmental Medicine Nos. 69/70. London: Spastics International Medical Publications/William Heinemann Medical Books.

— Blackwell RJ, Cusick G, et al. (1979) Ultrasound detection of brain damage in preterm infants. *Lancet* **1**: 1261–1264.

Papile L, Burnstein J, Burnstein R, Koffier H. (1978) Incidence and evolution of subependymal and intra-ventricular haemorrhage: a study of infants with birthweight less than 1500 g. *Journal of Pediatrics* **92**: 529–534.

Parmelee AH, Michaelis MD. (1971) Neurological examination of the newborn. In: Hellmuth J, editor. *The Exceptional Infant*. Vol 2. New York: Brunner Mazel. p 3–23.

Peiper A. (1928) *Die Hirntatigkeit des Sauglings*. Berlin: Julius Springer.

— (1963) Cerebral function in infancy and childhood. [Translation of the 3rd revised German edition by - Nagler B and Nagler H.] New York: Consultants Bureau.

Piper MC, Kunos I, Willis DM, Mazer B. (1985) Effect of gestational age on neurological functioning of the very low-birthweight infant at 40 weeks. *Developmental Medicine and Child Neurology* **27**: 596–605.

Polani PE, Mac Keith RC. (1960) In: André-Thomas, Chesni Y, Saint-Anne Dargassies S. (1960) *The Neurological Examination of the Infant*. Clinics in Developmental Medicine No. 1. London: National Spastics Society. Foreword, p 2–8.

Prechtl HFR. (1972) Pattern of reflex behaviour related to sleep in the human infant. In: Clements CD, Purpura DP, Mayer FE, editors. *Sleep and the Maturing Nervous System*. New York: Academic Press. p 287–301.

— (1977) *The Neurological Examination of the Full Term Newborn Infant*. 2nd ed. Clinics in Developmental Medicine No. 63. London: Spastics International Medical Publications/William Heinemann Medical Books.

— (1982) Assessment methods for the newborn infant, a critical evaluation. In: Stratton P, editor. *Psychobiology of the Human Newborn*. New York: John Wiley and Sons.

— (1990) Qualitative changes of spontaneous movements in fetus and preterm infants are a marker of neurological dysfunction. *Early Human Development* **23**: 151–159.

— Beintema D. (1964) *The Neurological Examination of the Full-term Newborn Infant*. Clinics in Developmental Medicine No. 12. London: Spastics International Medical Publications/William Heinemann Medical Books.

— Dijkstra J. (1960) Neurological diagnosis of cerebral injury in the newborn. In: ten Berge BS, editor. *Prenatal Care*. Groningen: Noordhoff.

— Fargel JW, Weinmann HM, Bakker HH. (1979) Postures, motility and respiration of low-risk preterm infants. *Developmental Medicine and Child Neurology* **21**: 3–27.

— Einspieler C, Cioni G, et al. (1997) An early marker for neurological deficits after perinatal brain lesions. *Lancet* **349**: 1361–1363.

Rennie JM. (1997) *Neonatal Cerebral Ultrasound*. Cambridge: Cambridge University Press.

Rollins NK, Morriss MC, Evans D, Perlman JM. (1993) The role of early MR in the evaluation of the preterm infant with seizures. *American Journal of Neuroradiology* **15**: 239–248.

Rutherford MA, Pennock JM, Dubowitz LMS. (1994) Cranial ultrasound and magnetic resonance imaging in hypoxic–ischaemic encephalopathy: a comparison with outcome. *Developmental Medicine and Child Neurology* **36:** 813–825.

— — Murdoch-Eaton DM, et al. (1992) Athetoid cerebral palsy with cysts in the putamen after hypoxic–ischaemic enecephalopathy. *Archives of Disease in Childhood* **67:** 846.

Saint-Anne Dargassies S. (1955) Méthode d'examen neurologique du nouveau-né. *Études Néonatales* **3:** 101–123.

— (1966) Neurological maturation of the premature infant of 28 to 41 weeks gestational age. In: Falkner F, editor. *Human Development*. Philadelphia: W B Saunders. p 306–325.

— (1977) *Neurological Development in Full Term and Premature Neonate*. Amsterdam: Elsevier/North Holland/Excerpta Medica.

Sarnat HB, Sarnat MS. (1976) Neonatal encephalopathy following fetal distress. *Archives of Neurology* **33:** 696–705.

Schulte FJ, Schrempf G, Hinze G. (1971) Maternal toxemia, fetal malnutrition and motor behaviour of the newborn. *Pediatrics* **48:** 871–882.

Touwen BCL, Bierman van Eendenburg MEC, Jurgens-van der Zee A. (1977) Neurological screening of full-term newborn infants. *Developmental Medicine and Child Neurology* **19:** 739–747.

Volpe JJ. (1978) Neonatal periventricular hemorrhage, past, present and future. *Pediatrics* **92:** 693–696.

— (1981) *Neurology of the Newborn*. Major Problems in Clinical Pediatrics No. 22. Philadelphia: W B Saunders.

THE NEUROLOGICAL ASSESSMENT OF THE PRETERM AND FULL-TERM NEWBORN INFANT

2nd Edition

Lilly MS Dubowitz, Victor Dubowitz, Eugenio Mercuri

Clinics in Developmental Medicine No. 148

Mac Keith Press

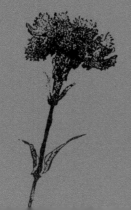

Distributed by

CAMBRIDGE
UNIVERSITY PRESS

ISBN 1-898-683-158

9 781898 683155

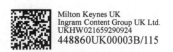